REIKI
and
MEDICINE

by

Nancy Eos, M.D.
Reiki Master

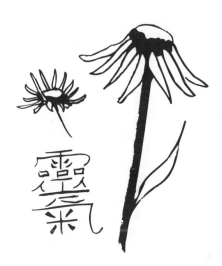

REIKI and MEDICINE

Copyright ©1995 by Nancy Eos, M.D.

Published by: Nancy Eos, M.D.

Computer graphics by: Glenn Lieding
                                          REBEARTH Inc.
                                          Ann Arbor, Michigan.

For information and additional books contact:

Nancy Eos, M.D.
P. O. Box 569
Grass Lake, MI 49240-0569
517-522-4880

International Standard Book Number 0-9644923-0-X
Library of Congress Catalog Card Number 95-90006
Published in the United States of America

Reiki and Medicine
Contents

Introduction

We first met Dr. Nancy Eos when she came to our Reiki I class. In the weeks following class, she frequently called to tell us of her experiences using Reiki in the emergency room. A seasoned ER doc, Nancy watched Reiki consistently help to reinstate the body's own healing balance in traumatic cases where the conventional medical approach alone could not account for the outcomes. It was thrilling to hear her stories; they provided evidence that blending this complementary healing modality with conventional medicine was making a difference.

Nancy had had no expectations regarding Reiki; yet as these events occurred, she observed them with an open mind. She documented the results, even though she could not always explain them because they showed up outside her medical paradigm. Her willingness to incorporate Reiki into her practice was evidence of her commitment and passion to provide the best care for her patients.

As you read this book you will encounter case histories that are outside mainstream Western medical thinking and perhaps outside your scientific framework. If you can suspend judgment and consider the possibilities that Reiki offers, you will open the door to a new medical paradigm. This integrated model contributes to the well being of both the medical professional and the patient. The doctor can use Reiki on himself to relieve stress as well as with his patients to alleviate pain, quiet fear and accelerate healing.

Dr. Eos is a leader in the exploration of mind/body medicine. We salute her pioneering spirit. It has been an honor and a privilege to train Dr. Eos as a Reiki Master and we look forward with delight to her experiences yet to come.

Reiki Masters Libby Barnett, MSW and Maggie Chambers

January 1995
Wilton, New Hampshire

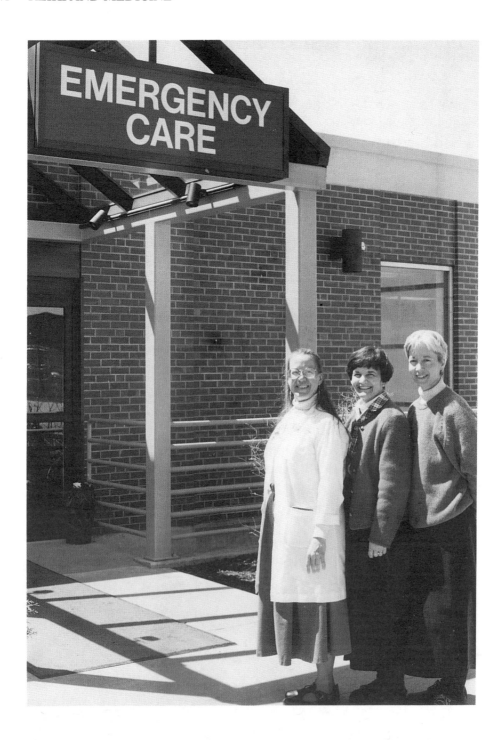

Forward

I became a happy, serene, medical doctor with Reiki. I chuckle inside knowing that I didn't have a whole lot to do with it all — it was Reiki — a universal love — an energy that we can tap into at anytime in any place for any reason in most any way and results happen.

The Reiki has not always produced predictable results but consistent results for the highest healing good. Marvelous results. Happenings not even able to be pre-conceived, not imagined. Lungs expand in spite of major chest trauma. Heart arrhythmias revert to normal sinus rhythm. Anger subsides to understanding. Narcotic addictions are satisfied with a mild sleeping pill. Strokes in progress reverse. Blindness releases to sight. Bleeding stops. Rigidity bends.

And I would not have believed any of this unless I had seen it for myself. Faith is something I have once I have it in my hand. I was given Reiki in my hands. I was skeptical but dared to try it, touch my patients, and then open to see whatever results might happen no matter how absurdly disconnected the cause and effect.

My life, my medicine and my career have all dramatically changed. I like it and I am happy. I went from the scientific mind of a university hospital medical school staff physician to the hands-on, frontline-medical practicality of a third world volunteer physician. Between both was a peak of earning money and acquiring all I ever wanted.

Reiki came to me two years ago while I was an emergency physician in a number of smaller hospitals. My daughter, and then I, were attuned to Reiki by Reiki Masters Libby Barnett and Maggie Chambers.

This book is a distillation of the numerous cases where Reiki and Medicine came together for me in the emergency room (ER). This book is for you about how to accept Reiki as a method of healing enhancement. It is about love. I can't imagine practicing medicine without Reiki.

February 1995   Nancy Eos
Grass Lake, Michigan

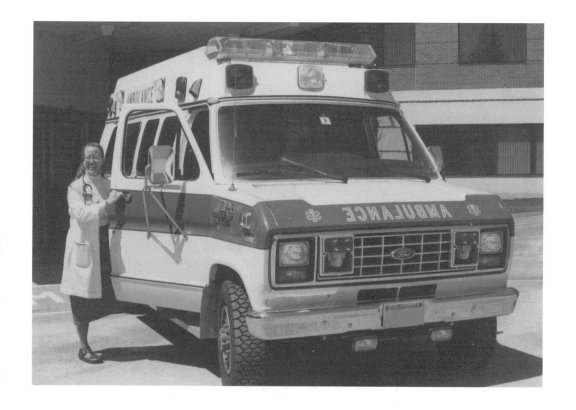

TRAUMA PATIENT
All Terrain Vehicle (ATV)

"Hi! I'm Dr. Nancy Eos," I say as I extend my hand to shake that of the Emergency Room (ER) patient. The registration clerk gave a call for a nurse to come up front to triage a patient in pain. The nurses are all busy and, being near the door, I came.

Reiki flows through hands.

He looks at me as if he is trying to care, trying to lift his right hand to shake the hand dangling in front of him. Pain overwhelms him. His chin goes down. He is only able to say, "I don't feel so good. I was testing my ATV and ran into a mudwall."

The placement of the hands begins Reiki.

I take his hand which has collapsed on the arm of the triage chair in an effort to hold himself up out of the pain. The touch begins Reiki. I grasp his wrist where it is and place my left hand on his shoulder allowing more touch for more Reiki. I lean in close to him and quietly ask what is happening as the Reiki is working.

Reiki is an unlimited energy flow from the universe through the attuned practitioner.

I learn a lot from this positioning. This is a sequence of positions I find gives me a wealth of information while immediately beginning to impart a bit of Reiki.

Reiki is a powerful compliment to traditional medicine.

The patient comes to the hospital Emergency Department indicating he is open to help. I assess his color, stance, and demeanor with my fifteen years of Emergency Medicine experience. Then I grasp

Permission is important to obtain.

By putting her hands on the patient, the attuned doctor is offering Reiki to the cells of the patient.

When a person's cells are intensely pulling in the Reiki, there is often an experience of heat for either the person or the Reiki practitioner.

The doctor's hands tell her that the cells are accepting of the Reiki.

hold of his body with my hands to let Reiki happen. I lean close to smell the breath, the body.

With this patient the heat I usually detect in my hands from the Reiki touch is not felt by me in his hand with the shake, nor in his shoulder in my other touch. I notice that he is twisting his neck a little as if he is having trouble getting words out.

My hands go to his neck. That is his hot spot. My hands feel hot. Not the electric hot plate searing heat like I felt with the 70 plus year old man who walked in late at night blue-lipped, drenched with diaphoresis and trying to die before my eyes because he was drowning in his own water in his lungs from his heart acting up. Not that immediate pain to the surface of my hands.

[By the way, that elderly man came around to pink and talking within ten minutes of continuing to put my hands on him for about 5-50 seconds every few minutes or so while the nurse and I began an intravenous line, started some oxygen, and connected the monitor.]

My ATV-slam-into-the-mudwall patient has a neck with slight swelling. There is no alcohol on his breath. He smells of fear. My hands feel the deep soft-tissue-is-hurting heat that I have found only a few people know they can detect. It takes practice to feel this tender heat. My left hand tends to feel it easier than the right but in some cases it is the opposite. I need to watch that more and see if there is a pattern.

Back to the trauma victim.

He continues to relate that he hurts in his neck and his left lower lateral ribs. I worry about his neck. The neck is for breathing. The trachea is the airway in the neck. It is the tube for oxygen. The body needs oxygen. The trachea is our access to control oxygen in the body. If a person blunt-traumatizes the front of his neck, he could have a fractured larynx, broken adam's apple or an altered vertebrae with swelling around the trachea. His life breath could be compromised quickly and the swelling block passages for emergency access. He could choke to death.

I let my hands stay around his neck — like a mother who is holding her son's face while looking at him and getting ready to kiss it to make it well.

I keep holding the neck, listening to him to try to relate to his pain, knowing that Reiki has the opportunity to be pulled in as long as I have my hands on him.

My eyes have not left his face. They, too, gather information. He is pink so oxygenating. He phonates well so the trachea is still intact. There are no bruises so I see no immediate bleeding or fractures.

He is young — 20's, healthy, generally happy — so good. He has city-outdoors clothes so might not have good judgment on trauma in the winter woods. He is about 5' 10", 160 pounds, average musculature.

Once attuned...
place hands...
allow Reiki.

There is nothing more
that is needed
to practice Reiki.

The emergency
assessment of trauma
can be analyzed even
while allowing Reiki.
No need to direct the
energy. No need to
concentrate
away from the
assessment.

Therefore, he will be easy to intubate or surgically install an emergency tracheostomy tube if necessary.

His breathing exchanges oxygen well but there is mild splinting of the left side. He may have hurt his left lung. There is no tracheal deviation so I doubt if his lung is collapsed right now.

"I place my hands for Reiki on every patient. Just a few seconds each time. A minute is a luxury. I try not to look too obvious. I just lay my hands somewhere in a neutral locality and then talk to the person."

All the muscles in his face and neck are working well. His hands and feet are working so his spinal column is okay — so far.

He appears to be walking and talking, beating and breathing okay, but he smells of fear and my hands are hot so he might be near collapse from significant blunt internal injury of neck, chest, and abdomen. If so, Airway and Breathing are of first importance. After the A and B, I will worry about Circulation.

"I hear your pain," I say. "We are going to help you right now. You don't have to wait. Hold on and we'll get a wheelchair to bring you back to a room. You don't have to walk any further." With that I release my hands from his neck and chin. Only two to three minutes have passed since I first saw the patient.

Two of our county's Emergency Medical Services (EMS) Paramedics are in the ER helping us out. They brought a patient in from an ambulance run, saw how busy we were and stayed on to help us. We have the best team in the state of Michigan of clerks, nurses, and EMS personnel as far as I am concerned. We have been in the newly expanded ER just one week. All our rooms are full. The intensity of the pathology is high today. Personnel is short. We are stretched thin in every way. It is disorganized in the new larger space but we are keeping on top of the most difficult cases.

This patient is one who could slip through the cracks. He doesn't yet look sick.

The nearest Medic grabs a wheelchair and transfers the patient from triage to our central working space. An angry father shouts from the waiting room that it isn't fair a person goes before his son. His family waits for two hours, his son has an earache. Their social services insurance is just as good as anyone else's payment.

[I saw the father later in the day. I shook his hand for the Reiki to flow. He calmed down and was shocked that the man he had complained about was the one who almost died. His anger quieted. But I am getting ahead of my story.]

I quickly make the rounds on the other patients to determine their status and make sure they are progressing well — awaiting labs, awaiting x-rays, private physicians called, no more vomiting blood since the Reiki of an abdomen, no worsening of a hot appendix since the Reiki, pulse

"I can't imagine practicing medicine without Reiki. With Reiki all I have to do is touch a person. Things happen that don't usually happen. Pain lessens in intensity. Rashes fade. Wheezing gives way to breathing clearly. Angry people begin to joke with me."

oximetry holding steady on an anemic woman who felt hot to the touch. We are busy.

When I come back to the trauma victim he is lying on the ER cart. They are sandbagging his neck into alignment. They are hooking him up to monitors. Everything looks fine. The nurses are beginning to look at me quizzically asking with their eyes — Why is he here? I don't say it is because his neck is hot to my hands.

In performing the initial trauma survey I feel every bone, look in every cavity, push on the ribs and belly, do a rectal exam. With each hand placement I think of Reiki. The neck is still hot to my hands. He flinches over the left lower lateral ribs but the abdomen is soft with no present problems detected. I hold my hands on him as long as I can. I leave the patient again. I have to. We are very busy.

Heat is not always detected, even in the places of active dangerous problems.

I check the orders: laboratory values, x-rays, electrocardiograms and oxygen status. We need these to transfer the patient to a trauma facility. I ask the clerk to call the larger hospital to start the transfer. The closest trauma facility is 90 minutes away by ground transport.

"Do you want me to have the helicopter team call you?" the Trauma ER Doc asks on the telephone.

I'm not sure the trauma patient needs the expense of a helicopter transport. However, if I say yes, I still have some time to reassess the patient and determine transport type later. I say, "Yes."

"I'll have them give you a call," he concludes.

I notice the neck cervical spine x-ray is being taken on the patient. The nurse has one intravenous (IV) line in place. I go in to re-examine him. He still phonates well, color good, vital signs stable, normal blood pressure, pulse, respirations, oxygenation, electrocardiogram is being taken.

Always support Reiki with standard medical and trauma protocol.

"You know, Dr. Eos, he was going 85 miles per hour when he rolled over," the nurse says. She happens to be the same nurse who worked with me on the female trauma victim where I first used Reiki.

"No, I didn't know. What else ?" The nurse doesn't know I already contacted the trauma hospital. She is trying to tell me he looks awfully good for the history she is obtaining.

"He was working on converting a jeep to an All Terrain Vehicle and in testing it out he hit a bank and rolled over. Probably put his neck and chest into the steering wheel. Then he bounced around on the ice. He says he was doing about 85 miles per hour when he crashed. Also, his left upper quadrant is a little tender."

My hands reach for the spleen area. Very tender. More tender than my last exam. Not a good sign. A broken spleen means he could bleed to death. I allow my hands to linger for a little extra Reiki.

Hands may merely linger but Reiki is flowing.

"Dr. Eos, the flight medic is on the line," the clerk says demanding I take my hands away from the patient to the phone. I am unable to go back to leave my hands on the spleen area for further Reiki. Could the little bit of Reiki be enough?

As I pick up the phone the x-ray technician slips the cross-table lateral cervical-spine film into my hands.

"Hello, can you fly?" I ask.

"We are getting the weather report as we speak. What do you have?" It is February up-State and fog or snow could keep them grounded.

"A 28 year old male in a 4-wheel drive ATV 85 miles-per-hour mudwall impact complaining of neck and left upper quadrant pain. I'm looking at the cervical spine film now and see a superior anterior chip fracture of C-6."

"How is his chest film? Is the mediastinum widening?" If the middle of the chest is getting larger on the x-ray then it means really bad things are happening inside the chest.

"We are getting the film right now."

"There is a weather front coming. We know we can get to you but we're not sure we can get back. We're still checking the weather report."

"That's okay because we are still putting in lines and foley and cutting the clothes off and immobilizing him. We have the Paramedics and rig here. When we get him ready, we have them here to immediately transport him if you can't come here because of the weather conditions."

"We'll call you back."

"Thanks."

The cardiology technician places the electrocardiogram tracing in front of me. The computer interpretation states normal but I see some small changes a young man should not have.

"Cardiac contusion," I say under my breath.

I head over to do more Reiki but another nurse catches me to come see a different patient.

So I was unable to get back to the 28 year old male for any significant Reiki. I did not have time to do distant Reiki. While I was busy with the rest of the emergency patients, the helicopter team came and quickly loaded the patient because of the weather front. He was gone before I knew it. I had wanted to keep placing hands for Reiki on his changing body conditions.

Seconds of Reiki may be enough.

The flight medic called later and said they had made it to the tertiary center hospital fine. The CT computerized tomography scan of the patient's neck was still inconclusive. On physical exam his abdomen was rigid. However, he was stable and the surgeons were watching him.

A minute is a luxury.

I use Reiki every day.

I place my hands for Reiki for every patient.

I see miraculous things happen. Positive changes which rarely happen in a certain deteriorating condition — happen regularly for me. They happen more and quicker the more I use Reiki.

With Reiki, miraculous things happen.

Positive changes happen regularly.

For instance: The summertime brings more people to the Emergency Department in the water wonderland of Michigan where I work. It gets extremely busy in the summer. It is hot.

People waiting for emergency care are kept from going out to play in the woods and on the lakes. They get grouchy waiting in the nonsmoking tiny waiting area. They have to tell the registering person what is wrong, then the triage person what is wrong, then they have to wait in an uncomfortable room until finally a person in a white coat comes in. They still hurt. No one has done anything to relieve the suffering. Instead, the sick and injured have had to suffer not only their condition, but the wait, the deprivation, the not being in control.

When I was first attuned to Reiki, I was curious to see how it would impact my ER work. I noticed that patients would become less angry after my hands were on them. No matter how angry I was in defensive reaction to their aggression, if I just placed my hands for Reiki the person became much less angry. Remarkably so.

So I began to put my hands on them sooner and sooner. And they began to calm down sooner and sooner.

For years I have extended my hand for a shake and to connect with the patient as soon as possible. However, it has only been since Reiki and noticing the difference in anger level that I now (1) walk in (2) put the charts down (3) turn to the patients and look them in the eye (4) extend my hand while I tell them my name (5) and then place my other hand somewhere on their body to begin the Reiki — on their hand, their elbow, their shoulder, or a hurting part of their body like their knee or face. Now, Reiki is a part of every patient contact.

I am asked if the dramatic healing and soothing changes are the result of Reiki or a placebo effect. Being an Emergency Physician, I am a master of the use of the placebo effect, but the results I see are beyond cognition, beyond the calming the mind can do for placebo. Reiki works for animals, for babies, for comatose individuals. Reiki is beyond placebo.

"What will my colleagues think of me believing in something like this?"

"What is 'this' that you are believing in?" I ask.

"You know, something that I don't understand."

"You don't have to understand it, just watch the results."

No matter how angry the person is -- if hands are placed for Reiki, the person becomes much less angry.

The doctor engages in the same procedures after attunement to Reiki as before. She notices the result of the contacts is now different.

Reiki is beyond the calming the mind can do for placebo.

*The patient's cells
dictate the process.*

*The doctor is like a
conduit tube.*

*The Reiki practitioner
does not deplete her
energy. Because of the
attunement by a Reiki
Master, only the
Universal Energy is
drawn upon with the
subsequent practice of
Reiki.*

*Reiki leaves energy in the
practitioner.*

"Does it always work?"

"Yes. Since the receiver's cells determine how much and where, the results are not always as the doctor would like to dictate, but Reiki always works."

"But what happens to ME when I do this Reiki? Won't I get tired having to put out all this healing energy?"

"No, the Reiki practitioner does not deplete her energy. Because of the attunement by a Reiki Master, only the Universal Energy is drawn upon with the subsequent practice of Reiki.

"The attuned doctor becomes like a conduit between the patient and a universal life energy. The doctor/practitioner moves beyond being a dispenser/manipulator of packets of medicinal energy. The doctor merely allows a flow through. The patient determines the amount and placement of the flow.

"Reiki always works. The receiver determines to what and what kind of extent. The receiver is in charge.

"I find the more active I am with Reiki, the more energized I become. The energy is especially evident at night in the ER. It is like some of the energy passing through me as a conduit hangs around and energizes me, too."

TRAUMA PATIENT
Motor Vehicle Accident (MVA)

Another trauma case in the Emergency Room (ER): A 21 year old female who had jumped out of her boyfriend's big, high, pickup truck going 30 miles per hour. She had not liked what her boyfriend was saying. Inebriated, he scooped her up, threw her in the front seat, and raced for our hospital. The nurses helped her onto a cart and wheeled her to the hallway. She was beating and breathing (meaning that she had a pulse and respirations). The nurses left her near the admitting desk while they finished completing care on the patients they were working with when they had been called away to assess the trauma victim.

I went over, listened to her screams that she could not breathe, and saw that she was very strong and active. She was thrashing about on the cart. She was pink. As usual, for the Reiki touch, I put both hands on her right side around my stethoscope as I listened to her chest. No breath sounds. My hands were hot.

There were no breath sounds on the right but I did hear a distant gurgling, like blood bubbling into a cavity. "Darn," I thought, "she may have a hemopneumothorax. It is the most probable injury in the chest with an MVA ejection injury."

Reiki can be used at any accident because you don't need special equipment.

Reiki can be used in the field before arrival of medical equipment.

Reiki can be used during transport.

Reiki can be used in the ER.

Reiki can be used with medical equipment in place.

Hands are placed for Reiki.

"The reason I instantly liked Reiki from the beginning is that I do not have to direct it, manipulate the patient, concentrate, etc. I like that idea. No identity with the result. Good or bad."

Hands are placed for Reiki.

Each place touched in the body has the opportunity to pull in the Reiki.

"I used the technique taught to me by my Reiki Master of always keeping one hand on the body while the other became situated ...so not to startle the life's energy pattern of the individual."

I felt for the trachea. It was deviated to the left. A deviated trachea is an indication there is tension against the remaining inflated lung. I felt the right rib cage. There were at least three ribs broken. This could be an indication of a flail chest. Bad news.

I rushed to the best nurse I could find and told her we probably had to insert a chest tube. I ordered the chest tray, oxygen, two intravenous lines, and the vital signs to be recorded every ten minutes. While I grabbed a needle in case I had to relieve a tension pneumothorax before we were finished with the chest tube preparations, I watched the patient and ordered the clerk to get the Emergency Helicopter Transport dispatcher on the telephone. I quickly documented the case on the chart, ordered an x-ray, talked to Emergency Medical Services (EMS) dispatch, and came back to the patient to reassess.

She was no worse.

I listened to her right lung again with my hands placed for Reiki on her chest while holding the stethoscope. No breath sounds. No gurgling. New finding. No more bleeding into the cavity.

I performed my secondary survey running my hands down her body touching and gently pushing every bone from skull through shoulders and pelvis to toes. Each place I touched as I assessed the integrity of the structures, the body had the opportunity to pull in the Reiki. I used the technique taught to me by my Reiki Master of always keeping one hand on the body while the other became situated so as not to startle the life's energy pattern of the individual.

The patient's cells pull the energy from the universe.

I listened to the heart and felt the belly. The heart sounded fine but she winced and groaned in the mid-abdominal region. She could also have an intra-abdominal injury. Bad sign.

The helicopter physician called back and said the helicopters were out on runs — could I wait or should they divert one to me? Just then the x-ray technician put the chest film up in front of me. Both lungs were expanded. The right lung had a funny appearance in the middle but it was definitely, totally expanded. A chest tube would not be needed. Was it the Reiki? Nothing else explained the discrepancy between the initial physical examination and this x-ray.

Amazing results can happen quickly.

I could see at brief glance at least three or four rib fractures. I said, "Wait a minute, let me reassess."

If she was still bleeding into the lung and possibly into the abdomen and she had a cardiac contusion (blow to the heart) — a high probability in any MVA with signifi-cant impact — she needed to be out of our little ER and into a trauma center STAT (as fast as possible)... and the nearest trauma center by ground transport for these major wounds was at least one hour away. She would never make it by ground.

Don't forget:
Place the hands for
Reiki.

Reiki always goes where
it is needed.

Reiki always supports
healing although it
may not be the cure we
hope for.

I dropped the phone without waiting to hear if it was okay with the other party. I went to the patient, listened, and kept my hands on her for Reiki while I found out what the latest vital signs were. No changes. She's holding her own. No tachycardia - fast heart beat which is a sign of bleeding.

I could even hear breath sounds now in BOTH lungs. The trachea was not deviated. I went back to the phone and told the receiving physician that the situation didn't look nearly as bad as it did in the beginning.

I didn't know what to say! I was amazed in mind-confusion. Could the Reiki make this person not need a trauma center? The woman had no health insurance. I was tempted to cancel the helicopter and have her transported by ground. Maybe she never had been as badly injured as I thought.

But I did send her to the trauma facility by helicopter. She had to wait hours for the transport. She did well but I worried about her the whole time she was in transit. We called the larger hospital later that evening. She did not go to surgery. She was stable enough to continue watchful waiting. A few weeks later I received a letter from the helicopter service. The woman did well but her discharge diagnoses included seven fractured ribs, a BROKEN STERNUM (the breastbone which is over the heart was broken), a cardiac contusion (a bruise of the heart), and a pulmonary contusion (a bruise of the lungs). Her abdomen had settled down during the overnight observation in the hospital intensive care unit.

I had doubted my pronouncement of the dire gravity of the situation with this case thinking it might have been overdoing it to send her to the trauma center by helicopter rather than the cheaper ground transport until a few shifts later when I experienced my second major Reiki case.

The nurse working with me on the second case gave me reason to dispel all doubt about Reiki being the cause of a re-expansion of a collapsed lung and cessation of bleeding into the chest. She told me she had seen the deviated trachea.
The reason she even brought it up is because she had not been able to believe what had happened to our 77 year old male patient — my second major Reiki case — so she asked me what I thought had happened. I told her it was Reiki.
She wanted an explanation of Reiki. Since I really didn't know and knew even less how to explain it, I told her about the 21 year old female MVA case.
That is when she told me that she had mentioned the deviated trachea to the nurse working on her with me. She had questioned why I or the flight team had not placed a chest tube prior to air transport.

Reiki is amazing.

"I found the changes would last for at least a few hours -- three to twelve -- and sometimes up to a few days.
"Perhaps my few seconds of the Reiki in the ER cured some patients. I don't know. They never came back.
"I was ALWAYS able to curb off the big problems
"--- at least until I transferred the patient and they arrived at the other hospital or until I left my shift in the ER."

Reiki is effective in all emergency situations whether in the ER, in the field, or home.

I told her that the x-ray had not supported the insertion of a tube. The x-ray had been taken after the Reiki. By the time the x-ray was taken, the trachea was not deviated. When the flight team arrived, no chest tube was needed.

When I come upon traffic accidents I stop and place my hands for Reiki. I try not to be in the way of the emergency personnel of the region. When they need me for my medical skills I stay on the scene with the patients and put my hands on the person. Otherwise, I stay in my car and employ the absentee Reiki to the situation.

HEART ATTACK PATIENTS
Myocardial Infarctions (MI)

MI Case #1

One time I transferred a 63 year old alcoholic diabetic man from our Emergency Room (ER) to the man's hometown hospital and the young doctor on the receiving end freaked. The electrocardiogram was obtained BEFORE I could get my hands on him for Reiki. AFTER Reiki, electrocardiogram changes consistent with a heart attack are often no longer present. In this case we did not obtain a second tracing after the Reiki.

Chest pain often dramatically diminishes after Reiki.

The first electrocardiogram showed some possible myocardial infarction (heart attack) changes. However, the chest pain had been present for days without purported change. I managed to get my hands on him for numerous short periods of time for Reiki. He had little chest pain after the Reiki.

Abnormal electrocardiogram tracings change after Reiki.

The blood for cardiac enzymes had also been drawn BEFORE the Reiki. The results were not back yet. However, I knew he needed an intensive care unit bed. So I made arrangements. The cardiac enzyme results came back after the patient was loaded in the transfer ambulance and on the road. We were trying to beat the winter weather front.

Reiki is love. Love is definitely for the heart.

"The quick, gentle healing without side effects changed me forever. I can't fathom staying in Medicine without using Reiki."

"It became widely realized that when people come to my ER they tend to get better unexplainably."

All heck broke loose. I had taken a second electrocardiogram which looked much better than the first. It did not support the diagnosis of an evolving infarction. The Reiki worked. I knew the patient would be okay for transport. The paramedics knew by now that regardless of the seeming condition of the patient on paper, if I said the patient would be okay during transport, he would. The paramedics, nurses and I had no problem with our transfer decisions regardless of the laboratory results. We treated the patient; not the laboratory values.

The enzymes were very elevated. They were off the wall. The patient was having a heart attack. I reported the enzymes and the electrocardiogram to the physician by fax since he couldn't talk to me on the phone right then.

He had the hospital's ER nurse radio the ambulance. The young, green physician ordered all sorts of acute heart attack medications. He put the orders through a three person relay: the doctor, the nurse, the dispatcher to the paramedic. None of the medicines were carried on the rigs. These were big time cardiac medications he was ordering. We heard this intense back and forth conversation on the radio in our ER. The doctor was worried that the patient wasn't going to make the trip. The paramedic was trying to say the patient was fine. The doctor was trying to find orders which would work for this patient enroute.

The paramedic was trying to help. Then the doctor told the ambulance to return to our ER because he was having a very bad heart attack. The paramedic informed him that they were in a snow storm and it was difficult to get to them let alone back to us.

The receiving physician did not know I had done Reiki. I knew the patient would be okay. The Reiki had worked. My hands had felt hot, cooled down on the patient, and the second electrocardiogram showed less acute changes. I was not worried.

The patient did do well. I called two days later. The young, concerned physician said the patient had indeed sustained an infarction, but there were no complications or trouble and no continual evolution since admission. He even said he, his private physician, was glad that the patient was there with him instead of remaining in our hospital that snowy night.

My lesson: I try to have the electro-cardiogram taken and the labs drawn AFTER the Reiki.

Electrocardiograms normalize and laboratory values are less dramatically abnormal when done AFTER Reiki.

Sticking to this time sequencing is less trouble for the patient, me as the ER Doc, and less trouble for the receiving doctor.

Sometimes the hands can detect subtle changes during Reiki.

Reiki often changes the course of events.

"Changing the sequence of events and adding Reiki became a conscious play for me."

MI Case #2

"I know medicine. I am a good diagnostician. But I don't like to treat anymore with all the side effects of medications and all the relapses when people don't take their breather space to change their illness to health."

Reiki always works. Place your attuned hands anywhere; Reiki goes where needed.

One time when I went to work, the physician supervisor came in for a few minutes to chastise me regarding the thrombolytic therapy protocol for recombinant tissue plasminogen activator that the hospital uses.

I didn't follow protocol on a chest pain patient during the last shift. He noticed it on peer review. Nothing bad had happened to the patient. That is not the point. I did not follow protocol. I was to follow protocol. I felt that I had good reasons for doing what I did. That didn't matter. Protocol is important.

This was the second time I had ordered thrombolytic therapy, it was made up, and it wasn't used. The thrombolytic medication is $5000 an injection. So I blew $10,000. Hummm. So did I say to him that I am having trouble using my theories about Reiki?? Trouble with my belief system about the good of conventional medicine??

I can hear my account now: "The first case had changes in the electrocardiogram because it was taken before I had a chance to allow Reiki to work. By the time I finished placing my hands for Reiki, she had no more chest pain except when I pressed on her costochondral joints. I decided not to give her a high powered drug with many side effects since she had a reason for the remaining pain. I knew the Reiki was enough and the patient would be okay." Do you think he could take that to the hospital committee as the explanation for not giving the thrombolytic medication? Not a good idea.

In the second case the electrocardiogram was taken AFTER a LOT of Reiki. This patient had a classic chest pain history for myocardial infarction with NO changes on his electrocardiogram. Hummm.

Reiki is a powerful compliment to traditional medicine.

Note the order: I had seen electrocardiographic changes on the initial monitor strip indicating a possible heart attack in evolution. Not good. His history was classic for a heart attack in evolution. Not good. I called for thrombolytic therapy. Good — assuming the tests would support this by the time the thrombolytic medication was drawn up, mixed and ready for injection. I placed my hands for Reiki. Good — period.

THEN I ordered the electrocardiogram and cardiac enzymes to support the initiation of the thrombolytic therapy. I was sure the tests would support the thrombolytic therapy decision.

Just as we were to give the thrombolytic medication to the patient through the intravenous line, the electrocardiogram tracing was normal and the STAT enzymes came back normal. The patient had no more chest pain. I ended up not giving the $5000 medication.

"I was still learning how to blend Reiki and Medicine.

Test results become less alarming.

The usual course of events change.

The patient's usual responses are altered.

"I was not in control."

So I was reprimanded for not giving thrombolytic therapy in the first case and for having it made up needlessly in the second.

These cases were within the first month or two after I was attuned to Reiki. I was still learning how to blend Reiki and Medicine.

In the first case Reiki BEGAN after the tests were taken. In the second case Reiki began BEFORE the tests.

... And both patients did well.

This phenomenon of test results being less severe after Reiki happened regularly but only these two times caught the attention of others. I became frustrated with the course of most events. I wanted to be in charge. It was clear if I allowed Reiki into the situation, I was not in control. The patient's usual response processes to the disease or to the therapies were altered. I could no longer predict outcomes. The statistical outcomes studied into every part of my emergency physician brain were useless. Predictability of responses is what any physician counts on. It is our ace-in-the-hole. We always know what will probably happen. We count on it.

So... I began to place my hands to give Reiki to the patient BEFORE the electrocardiogram and have the blood drawn AFTER the electrocardiogram. If the electrocardiogram showed changes, I would allow Reiki again before the blood work was drawn for the laboratory tests. By choosing this sequence of Reiki BEFORE orders, I had less positive changes of the electrocardiogram and cardiac enzymes. Even if the electrocardiogram showed some heart attack changes, I would order the electrocardiogram repeated before prescribing the thrombolytic therapy. If there are no acute electrocardiogram changes then, per protocol, no thrombolytic therapy is to be given.

By sequencing Reiki BEFORE orders, less and less invasive procedures were required.

As a result, I have not given any more thrombolytic medication. It's been over a year now. I manage to slide under the protocol guidelines for the mandatory administration of thrombolytics every time just by manipulating when I order the tests in relation to when I place the hands for Reiki. And the patients do fine. This is the most important thing. The patient does well.

And, most importantly... the patient does well.

If I reported the patient to the receiving physician before the laboratory tests and the blood for the tests were drawn after the Reiki, not even the laboratory values supported the dire distress the patient was in on admission to the general county hospital ER. The receiving specialists began to think I was crying wolf. They began to think I was over reactive. But word slowly got around through the nurses and family of the patients that truly, the patient was doing poorly when they went to the ER but turned around quickly while there.

Reiki complements traditional medical techniques.

Reiki is not a magic pill; it never overrides the ultimate destiny or patient choice.

"My hands-on-healing technique I used before Reiki attunement would seem to stop up in me. I would get what my patient had. Then I learned Reiki. Now I am a compassionate straw which merely allows the universal energy to flow to those who take it. Some of the energy rubs off on me and I actually glow from inside out after a Reiki contact."

I often tried to leave a reason for the quick turn around. I gave an antacid for chest pain and assign the disappearance of the pain to the medication even though the pain began receding before the liquid was taken.

I gave instructions to breathe out and in very slowly and long to the collapsed lung patients while I would listen and place hands for Reiki. I told them it must be the new breathing that caused the pain to go away and the lung expand.

Patients like explanations. They want to know what is going on. Should I say, "Oh, just Reiki." Not. Not always a good idea.

But what about the ethics of taking away the patient's pain?

What about the possibility of masking an important problem?

What about the possibility of recurrence at a time when they cannot get back to the ER? What if the patient ignores the pain the next time because it turned out to be nothing this time?

The patient is the one who controls the effects of the Reiki. In watching the responses I have found that when a patient makes a significant discovery or a life-style change, their reason for being in the ER disappears.

I have seen patients relapse — often. But does that mean we should not try to aid them as fully as we can at the time that we see them? If we are supposed to do nothing, then we should not give oxygen to one who smokes. They will just go back and smoke some more necessitating more need for oxygen. If we are to do nothing, then we should not be giving allergy mist treatments to asthmatics who have pets they are allergic to.

I tell the patient their body is speaking to them. It does not matter the outcome or how bad or less bad the diagnosis of their pain is: Their body is trying to say they are hurting someplace.

PAY ATTENTION.

Reiki brings energy from outside the system to help the emergency situation.

My theory is that once the patient hears the message and begins to change, the patient's body is lagging behind — stuck in the body emergency situation. Reiki brings energy from outside the system to help. Once the acceptance for change is there, Reiki provides energy to help the change happen.

Relapses are normal. Reiki also helps relapses. Relapses need self-Reiki. Repeated Reiki by a practitioner also helps. The practitioner need not be a physician.

RESPIRATORY PATIENTS
Shortness of Breath (SOB)

Back to the second major Reiki case: A 77 year old male came to the Emergency Room (ER) at two o'clock in the morning accompanied by his wife. He was drenched. The clerk asked, "Is it raining out?"

The laboratory technician said, "Page the Nurse overhead STAT. He's blue and can't breathe. That is perspiration."

The nurse rushed in and commanded, "Get Dr. Eos in here immediately."

I came running in to see an elderly man, sweating, cool-clammy skin, mildly cyanotic, and unable to speak because he was working so hard at trying to breathe. I noticed his wife. I tried to get some history from her while I listened to his lungs.

No wheezing, no breath sounds, his chest was tighter than a drum. Did his life-threatening condition begin suddenly or slowly? Did he have a history of this behavior previously? Was the answer to his relief in attacking (1) a lung problem of tightness which was constricting his mechanical ability to breathe, or (2) a heart problem of inability to pump the blood which backed up the fluid in a short time totally filling his lungs. The treatments are exactly opposite. Treating one wrongly would aggravate the other.

Positive changes which rarely happen in a certain deteriorating condition -- happen regularly with Reiki.

I turned to his wife for the history. She was concerned about the condition of her husband and was acting inappropriately. It appeared like she had a mild dementia perhaps Alzheimer's disease. Still no history. The patient couldn't talk either. No old chart here from medical records.

There must be an intention. Reiki must be thought of then place the hands.

I realized I had not yet put my hands on the patient to allow for Reiki. While I was trying to think and decide which way to go with little information, I placed my hands on his right shoulder and right forearm.

Immediately I felt heat under my hands and reflexly began to withdraw. It was like putting them on an electric griddle. But I logically knew that he should be cool because of the blueness and the perspiration. Sweat was rolling off of him from everywhere.

"It was like putting my hands on an electric griddle."

It is then that I dramatically realized: Reiki works. Without a doubt. Something was going on between my hands and his body. I was not controlling it. There was nothing to do or not do. I kept my hands there for about 50 seconds as I thought in my medical mind how to get the patient out of this predicament.

There is nothing more to do or not do.

The nurse had placed oxygen on him. His oxygen saturation was registering in the low 80's. Bad news. I told her to concentrate on the IV (intravenous line for fluid

Reiki means universal life force - the healing, loving, creative energy that interpenetrates all of creation.

administration into the vein). I told the clerk to call for an electrocardiogram and chest x-ray.

I released my hands to start writing on the chart and try again to get some history from the wife. I was restless with that activity, though, and found myself drawn back to placing my hands on him. There was still a violent heat-like reaction.

In all, I had my hands on him four or five times over the next ten minutes. We finally gave some medication to reduce the fluid in the lungs (furosemide) by injecting it into the IV once the IV was placed but it takes a while for it to help. However, he began to reverse right before our eyes within that ten minutes even before the IV was established.

He had been close to coding (a cardiorespiratory arrest where the heart and the lungs stop working). Even if he hadn't been quite that advanced in his pathology, he was sorely in need of oxygen and had all the signs for immediate intubation (an airway placement to allow oxygen to be forced into the lungs).

But while I was getting ready for those maneuvers, I had placed my hands. They felt a contact heat. The patient bega Within ten minutes he was out of the emergency and breathing enough to tell me what had happened. He could talk again. He didn't have to be intubated. His oxygen saturation was now at 92%.

A miracle.

The patient's cells were enthusiastically drawing in the Reiki producing intense heat.

Reiki often changes the usual course of events.

Amazing results happen quickly.

When a person's cells are intensely pulling in the Reiki, there is often an experience of heat for either the person or the Reiki practitioner.

"Still doing very well at work. Still using my hands -- Reiki -- and getting great responses. Now the nurses and clerks are asking for Reiki. It has become a joy to go to work. I get excited driving toward the hospital just wondering how I will discover Reiki next."

Often the person displays a sudden significant change in health well before medical procedure interventions.

The more severe and sudden the problem, the more dramatic the response to Reiki.

He said later that he had overexerted during the day by going up and down his stairs at home a few too many times. After watching a ball game on television, he lay down to sleep. Just as he was falling asleep, he felt like the blood was running out of his fingers and his feet. Then he could not get his breath. He struggled with the sensations, awakened his wife, and the 75 year old lady drove him to the ER because they did not want to disturb the Emergency Medical Technicians so late at night. By the time he got here he was blue and drenched in sweat from the work of trying to breathe.

My guess is that he had his heart stop and fluid backed up in his lungs. He was on one medication for the heart for the last six years. No other medications. No other problems.

Note: In many cases the person displays a sudden significant change in health well before medical procedure interventions. In many cases the person has a strong desire to be well but cannot muster enough innate strength to complete the process alone. In many cases a doctor attuned to the universal life energy touched another individual allowing a flow of Reiki.

Trauma patients and medical patients in dire straits generally respond readily and quickly to the Reiki. The more severe and sudden the problem, the more dramatic the response.

Chronic Obstructive Pulmonary Disease

The paramedics rolled in the ER with a 63 year old female with chronic obstructive pulmonary disease. She was blue. Tight wheezes. Still alert. Pulse oxygenation reading at 65% which is very very low. Not a good picture.

"My doctors say I could die anytime," she stated. She had end-stage lung disease. She had been released from another hospital just two days previously. They gave her no hope for living during the next attack. She decided to visit her family before she died. The excitement of the extended family was a bit much for her. She carried her home oxygen unit with her at all times. She still smoked cigarettes in spite of the use of the oxygen unit.

"Well, not today. Okay?" I responded as I placed my hands and let the Reiki unfold. She looked close to having a respiratory arrest right that very second.

"Okay," she responded — much to my surprise.

And she must have meant it because she began to perk up a bit. His gray color turned to light reddish-blue. Maybe the Reiki of a few seconds was working already.

She wanted to go back to her home hospital. It was hours away by ambulance. There was a good chance she would not make it. She refused to be intubated before

"I had a headache the whole shift. Even while placing hands for Reiki. The cases became dramatically better anyway. I don't have to be in a good mood to have the Reiki work. This is important to me. My headache is my problem, not the patient's."

The patient is the active participant in Reiki.

transport. Intubation is the placement of a tube down the throat through the mouth to help the patient breathe better.

I placed my hands for Reiki. I touched her at least fifteen times over forty minutes and then agreed to the transfer. The ambulance personnel were apprehensive but they also placed a lot of trust in my judgment. They agreed to transport her without the usual tube placement in this kind of case for assured breathing.

I knew she had accepted a great deal of Reiki but I was still apprehensive. If she coded enroute (cardiorespiratory arrest) I had no defense to accusations of deviation from standard medical care.

It was the end of my shift. I had two hours to drive home. I placed my hand for absentee Reiki for her while I drove all the way back home.

I called the hospital. She tolerated the ambulance trip well. The receiving nurses wanted to know why she had to be admitted, since she looked so good and pink. They knew her from a previous hospitalization. She was rarely oxygenating well enough to have pink mucus membranes.

The nurses receiving her wondered if I knew what I was doing. They wondered if I knew when a patient was okay or not okay. Was I a physician who just cried wolf to get patients admitted somewhere?

The medics showed them her pulse oxygenation statistics before admission to our ER. The nurses agreed that before

"I found the changes from Reiki would last for at least a few hours - three to twelve - and sometimes up to a few days."

"Often, this breather was all the person needed to continue toward health."

"Not good for my ego. But better to look like I cry wolf than to have somebody croak."

transport she must have been doing poorly even for her.

This question of my competance by the receiving doctors and nurses who regularly saw a healthier patient than I described was not good for my physician ego. But better to look like I cry wolf than to have somebody croak.

She did well in the other hospital for the first twelve hours. Then she stopped breathing. They tried to restart her heart and lungs by coding her three times before she died the next day. She had the opportunity, though, to have the rest of the family say goodbye.

A person's will and destiny always dictates the final outcome.

Pneumothorax cases

Though I have been the attending physician for three pneumothorax (lung collapse) cases since I was attuned to Reiki, I haven't yet had to insert a chest tube after Reiki of the lungs.

The emergency conditions persist but the severity is much less after Reiki.

One lung collapse case where I couldn't hear any breath sounds on the affected side before Reiki... was documented at 15% on the x-ray... the x-ray was after the Reiki. Fifteen to twenty percent is about the percentage when a chest tube should be ordered. The collapse being at 15%, the chest tube was not mandated by standard medical procedure. Therefore, I didn't place one. Instead, I placed my hands for more Reiki.

Every patient becomes a discovery with Reiki.

The other two pneumothorax cases resolved before my very eyes. The deviated trachea came back to midline in both. A deviated trachea is an indication that the trachea has been pulled to one side of the chest because the lung collapsed.

These findings are just like the nurse described for my motor vehicle accident MVA trauma patient. At first look the trachea is deviated. After Reiki, it is not.

So, like the 42 year old male with a heart attack who was better without the usual heavy drugs with multiple side effects — a 23 year old male with a pneumothorax became better without the usual invasive procedures. He still had the emergency condition but the severity was much less than before I placed my hands for Reiki.

Conditions become better for the patient, for the doctor, and for the staff.

Just a bit of placement of the hands for Reiki — that's all I did — and conditions became better for the patient, for me, and for the staff while in the ER.

CARDIOPULMONARY RESUSCITATION
Arrest
(CPR)

One morning at the general county hospital we had a 67 year old male in full arrest who collapsed at the check out counter of a store in the corner of the county. He was unresponsive and remained a straight line on the cardiac monitor showing he had no heartbeat until just outside the Emergency Room (ER) door. I headed out to see the patient. I opened the back door of the ambulance and grabbed hold of the foot of the patient to allow the Reiki to begin. He immediately converted to sinus cardiac rhythm -- regular spontaneous heartbeat.

He was still blue, no pulse. We brought him in the ER heart room and I touched him as often as I could. The paramedics were still performing cardiopulmonary resusitation since there was no pulse. As soon as we transferred him to the ER cart and checked for a pulse, he had one. Full arrest with long down time and he came back to sinus rhythm with a pulse. Unreal. He pinked up. Unreal. Reiki?

He was a full arrest, no hope. The ambulances are stationed near the hospital in the center of the county. It had taken the medics about 20 minutes to get to him where he collapsed. It took the team another 45 minutes or so before they were at our back door.

"I place my hands for Reiki with every patient. I touch every patient. Just a few seconds each. A minute is a luxury."

With Reiki there is no need to direct energy, manipulate the patient or concentrate.

"It is exciting going to work now. I wonder how Reiki will work next."

We are talking about one hour of straight line on the monitor and NO spontaneous heart beats. It could not have been a mistake of overcall on the part of the emergency personnel. These were excellent licensed paramedics well trained and with years of experience.

After listening to the radio banter between the EMS unit and the base station physician, we were going to assess this patient, note that all the advanced cardiac life support ALS protocol had been followed and stop the code once he arrived at our doors. We were going make the assessment in the ambulance so that he would not be charged an ER visit. But he changed for the better. So we continued care.

Because there is no intensive care unit and no respirator in our little hospital, we sent him on to the bigger hospital for further care. Interesting.

He died nine hours later. We had no other knowledge surrounding the events of his death. His family was able to visit and say good bye while he was in the intensive care unit. He did not recover consciousness. His body was able to give some organs for transplant. Interesting.

The course and outcome of a case is often different than what we had wished.

Another ambulance call on the radio. I went over near the radio which sits on the counter next to the admitting clerk. I clutched the counter under my hands and asked for Reiki and the best highest healing to the patient they were reporting about. Ten minutes later they said over the radio that the patient was better. The person decided not to come to the ER by ambulance. Interesting.

CHILD ABUSE PATIENT
Child Abuse And Neglect
(CAAN)

Nothing affects an Emergency Room (ER) like a child abuse case. Nothing. Not even death. Death is so final. A child in an abusive situation is not final. I'm so glad I have Reiki now.

"I'm so glad I have Reiki now."

One weekend at general county hospital we were sent a protective services case. These referrals were usually cases with suspected sexual child abuse issues. As I always do, I watch the nurses when a highly emotionally charged issue is to enter the ER. There was the usual intensity and each person was keeping personal reactions out of the workplace. We were already full and busy in the ER.

I looked at the chart of the patient wondering if memories from my own childhood would come flooding back. No problems yet. The daily self-Reiki during the past year helped immensely to heal these memories.

Daily self-Reiki helps to heal memories.

I placed my hands on the chart to begin Reiki while reading what the nurses had written. I asked for Reiki to the situation through the chart and said thank you under my breath in respect to Reiki. I requested Reiki to come to me and this child in this exam.

Ask for Reiki to the situation.

Sometimes hands become hot while resting on an inanimate object connected to a Reiki situation.

My hands were not particularly hot while resting on the chart. Sometimes my hands become hot while resting on an inanimate object connected to a Reiki situation.

I first noticed this diagnostic help when I went to the counter by the Emergency Medical Services EMS radio to receive incoming calls. I made it a practice to place my hands directly on the counter by the radio. When bad cases were to be transported to my ER, my hands often felt a little swollen and a burning sensation arose in the palms and spread through the fingers. At other times I could immediately feel the burning when I picked up the chart of the next ER patient to be seen.

Good, I thought. This is probably another disheveled home and not a case of outright physical abuse.

I headed to Room 4.

We had been quiet in the ER from 8am when I began my shift until almost 3pm. Then within the course of an hour we filled all ten rooms and still had four people in the waiting area to be brought back as soon as possible. Beds 5, 6, 7, and 8 were all admissions to our tiny thirty bed hospital. I hadn't yet been able to phone any of their private physicians. Much paperwork left to do. The lab work was not back yet for evaluation.

All four patients to be admitted were stable. However, I had a gut-level not-good-feeling about Bed 5. He was a 76 year old male with three days of epigastric abdominal distress changing today to heaviness extending into the chest. He denies that the heaviness is chest pain. He is youthful appearing. A go-getter. He went to town with the great-grand kids today. He wasn't feeling well before he left but he didn't want to disappoint the grandchildren. He so much enjoyed being with them. So he went. So now he is in my ER... with my hands burning when I touch him... with rales half-way up each lung... probably congestive heart failure... failure for his heart to keep up with his body and his mind. He smiles but now and again he takes a deep breath and a look of concern fleets across his tiny drawn face.

Once the acceptance for health is there, Reiki provides the energy to help the change happen.

I scurry past him and on to Room 4 while thinking about Reiki and knowing I probably don't need as much Reiki for them as for me. I am the one in this situation who needs the Reiki. I have trouble with child abuse cases. I get very personally involved.

"I probably don't need as much Reiki for them as for me."

She is sitting on the rolling doctor's stool. 12 years old. 4 feet 11 inches. 85 pounds. Pretty clean. Smile on face. No obvious bruises. Obviously no pain. Ready to cooperate. No anger issuing forth towards me or Dad who was the only other one in the room. Normal child. Going to be a normal exam.

I looked at the father. He sat toward the edge of the chair. Cane in right hand. One of those hardwood self-made canes. He was tall and very heavy with a body profile a pear shape — so the cane was thick around. He was filthy.

He had on jeans-coveralls that didn't look worked in — no mechanics grease, no farmers soil — just worn a long time. His flannel shirt was rolled up at the sleeves revealing a very dirty long sleeved under-shirt. His face was projecting sweetness and smiles at me which crossed paths with lines of anger when I mentioned the wait he must have had to endure just because an agency wanted his daughter to be seen by me.

His countenance flitted back from anger to apparent understanding and a let's-get-on-with-it attitude. I turned my attention back to the child/young adult. The girl was the patient — not the dad. Was this child abused? Was any medical evidence available? There didn't appear to be.

Reiki is drawn through the practitioner.

"What happened?" I said as I looked into her eyes, smiled, and put my hands under her chin to feel the cervical lymph nodes but allowing the touch to be more like a Mom's who is about to kiss a child and make it well. I was thinking Reiki. My touch for the exam allowed Reiki.

"Oh, I was crying in school so they sent me in here... but I fell, you see, at school...

No need to direct energy.
No need to force results.
No need to identify with the outcome of Reiki.

"I was running backwards and fell... so later I was crying a little and they sent me here," she said.

"Oh," I said — unconcerned with the story and concentrating on the physical exam. I knew my hyperacute senses for child abuse would nudge me in its own time IF it was there. No need to concentrate on that. I make it a habit to concentrate fully on physical hard-fact findings while I keep the patient busy talking by asking a few simple questions.

"I make it a habit to concentrate fully on physical hard-fact findings while I keep the patient busy talking -- and place hands for Reiki."

Alert and Appropriate.

Well Developed Well Nourished Female in No Acute Distress.

"Well have you had any recent cold, sore throat,..."

Head Eyes Ears Nose Throat: clear. Neck: supple without lymphadenopathy.

"...fever,..."

Spine: non-tender without costo-vertebral angle CVA tenderness. Lungs: clear. Heart: regular rhythm without murmur.

"...nausea, vomiting,..."

Abdomen: soft, good bowel sounds, non-tender.

"...constipation, diarrhea, burning when you pee?"

Neurological: within normal limits and strong for age. Deep tendon reflexes normal. Extremities: full range of motion without edema. Skin: without bruises but abrasions on right upper outer hip with well healing tiny scabs. Genitals: normal. No bony tenderness.

"No."

"Any other recent problems?"

"No."

On the belly exam she had taken a little longer to lay down and get back up off the examining table but I thought it was reluctance at exposing herself in a flat position even though she remained clothed throughout the exam.

Nothing else abnormal about the exam. The chart said: "Father backed over daughter in driveway c/o right shoulder and thigh."

Yes. Read that again: FATHER BACKED OVER DAUGHTER IN DRIVEWAY COMPLAINS OF RIGHT SHOULDER AND RIGHT THIGH. 12 year old girl. Van driven. Doesn't take a bright mind to tell something's wrong with this picture. Also doesn't take much common sense to hear that the story being told to me about the school "fall" is not in reality a major issue in this exam room at this time. I have been with the girl for about ten minutes and neither the Dad nor the girl has offered an iota of information about the van incident. What gives here?

A concerned parent with nothing to hide would go straight to the accusation of running a child over with a van. Right? Even if they were ashamed, a loving parent would want to know from the first doctor seeing the child since the accident that the child was physically okay. Right?

The purported accident happened five days previously. I am the first medical person to check the child. Something is wrong with this picture. But the child checks out okay. She is voicing no complaints, she is showing no anger toward her father. My hands do not get hot touching this child. Something does not fit right in this puzzle. In fact, nothing fits. As far as I can tell though, all is settled within this room.

But somewhere from a deep place inside of me I felt an order to get x-rays. So I did. No real indication other than the chart that said 'Father backed over daughter in driveway, complains of right shoulder and right thigh.' I ordered the shoulder and the pelvis. The pelvis because the radiograph would include both hips which are a little difficult to fully palpate on manual exam. Both thighs were nontender to physical examination. Also, since the shoulder and thigh had been mentioned by social services on the referral, these films would be the best evidence for the juvenile court in defense of the family against any community or school charges should they be falsely accusing this family of abuse.

I thought no more of the discrepancies until I was reading the x-rays. Her films were in the third folder to be read. I was hurrying through the batch nonstop. I was interrupted by a nurse asking questions about another patient. I continued to read films. She was startled when I dropped my mouth, sucked my breath in and pointed to the pelvic bone fracture. She gasped.

"Who is that?" she asked.

"The patient in four," I said.

"But she doesn't seem to be in pain even when she walks."

"Precisely. This child has to be in much more pain than she is showing."

The break in the bone was entirely through the right superior pubic ramus with a significant amount of displacement.

YOU ARE SO FORTUNATE IF YOU GET TO FEEL AND SHOW PAIN. IT MEANS YOU ARE SAFE TO FEEL. FEEL PAIN. HOW CAN YOU FEEL JOY IF YOU CAN'T EVEN FEEL PAIN?

...often times things are not as they appear to be...

I am trying to say that often times things are not as they appear to be. I have found it true so far on many case follow-ups that Reiki always works. It always does something somewhere. It may not produce an outcome which I thought I wanted to happen... BUT LOVE DOES START SHOWING THROUGH.

Reiki always works.

So I went back into the room. I had the patient sit on the exam table. I watched as she moved up into position. She favored the right leg in getting up onto the table and down again. I knew what was the source of her twinge from pain. The x-ray had told me. It shouted out the whisper from the limp of the child. The secret was no longer secret. I knew she had to hurt 20 times more than she was displaying to me. The x-ray said so. The x-ray demanded attention. The child avoided attention.

She laid herself back on the table to be examined.

She had to hurt... the x-ray...

I laid my hands gently on her hips. I thought about Reiki. No heat. I squeezed. No response.

"Did that hurt?" I asked.

"No," she answered. A smile was on her face.

I went over the specific bone which was broken. No heat felt by the Reiki touch. I pushed. One part of one of her arms winced. She still had the plastic smile on her face.

"Did that hurt?" I asked.

She answered, "No."

Hands don't always become hot. If Reiki is effective as a diagnostic tool, why didn't the hands get hot near the pelvis? Reiki is not predictable. Perhaps it was not 'safe' for the cells of the child to pull in Reiki.

Rage welled up inside me. I threw a glance at the father... the father who had BACKED OVER DAUGHTER IN DRIVEWAY. I wanted to rake him over the coals so that he might get a tad of the pain his daughter was not expressing.

I recognized my anger. I allowed Reiki to myself.

Out came the words, "Your daughter has a broken pelvis."

Nothing more.

No rage.

Self-Reiki is also not predictable.

I continued holding my hands on myself. No longer did I have the anger. I was surprised at the compassion I felt — for him, for the child, for me and for the world. The Reiki was working on me. Had Reiki worked for the child?

Reiki over a period of time helps adults through their own personal child abuse issues.

I have found that regular periodic sessions of Reiki over a period of time has helped adults through their own personal child abuse issues. I've seen some people diagnosed as multiple personality disorder come barging into my home, fly across the room and crumple near me begging for a little hands-on Reiki. Then they sobbed and sat there while we let the Reiki work. People who couldn't even tolerate a hug the year before. Sometimes stories would spill out, more often just sobs would come.

All the child-abused people eventually became calmer, happier, and freer to be integrated to one self. This happened over the short but intense periods I would get to intermittently give them Reiki.

Every patient became a discovery with Reiki.

Those positive results were in long term usage of Reiki -- thirty sessions twenty minutes each. What about this child? No one else in general county hospital has been attuned to Reiki at this time. This child may never receive more Reiki. By placing hands and allowing Reiki, have I given hope where I should not?

I think even a little Reiki is better than no Reiki. Also, when used, Reiki always works somewhere, someway. As the practitioner I may not see the results or may not recognize the change immediately. Too, my wishes for certain conclusions may not allow me to see the highest healing good.

"I hadn't realized how scared I was... until the fears were gone... with Reiki."

I left the room.

I felt the tension in the ER. Word had spread that the tiny girl in Room 4 had a displaced pelvic fracture. The nurses were waiting for my reaction. Nurses often key into the mood of the physician. We were full of new admits. We had every room full. We didn't have time for some ER Doc to rant and rave just because of some injustice in this world.

I went into the Doctor's dictating room and put my hands on my head for Reiki. I only had a fraction of a minute for it before I was called away to the phone and then to the many other emergencies.

All went well for awhile after that. I was able to put the personal emotional reactions about child abuse aside until later after the ER was completely cleared out.

The child was admitted to the hospital for further tests. The Protective Services worker came and was questioning the nurses in the ER. He and I went into the back room and talked. I found myself getting angrier and angrier. So I placed hands to allow Reiki to myself.

Suddenly I felt a relaxation come over me. I stopped in mid-sentence, looked at the Social Worker and said, "You know, it doesn't matter if you get the correct evidence you need for your court case. What matters is that the Dad and the Child both know that we care. That we are here. And that someone will continue to be here for each of them."

I had found that as an ER Doc I had needed to put up walls around my emotions to keep from getting caught up and dragged down while flitting between patients in the ER. There are big cases, lots of emotions, life and death issues, and many triggers for past personal injustices.

"No matter what happens... with Reiki... it is so much fun these days to treat people. I love being a doctor. I am learning a lot about myself."

The practitioner may not see the results or may not recognize the change immediately.

"...holding my hands on myself... I was surprised at the compassion I felt... for me and for the world..."

Since I learned Reiki I am able to rush between the emotions faster still being empathetic and feeling love. The intense feelings which promote shutdown and the triggers of those automatic protective reactions are noted sooner. I recognize the trigger event, thank the opportunity for emotional growth, and set aside the blockage to happiness. I continue to function and to love — me and the patient in the immediate situation.

"...with Reiki I continue to love -- me and the patient -- in the immediate situation."

Did the Reiki do anything to calm me in this situation? the child? the Dad? the ER? the nurses?

I think so. Yes, Reiki helped closure for all of us.

The attuned physician thought of Reiki, bothered to apply hands for Reiki, and things got better. The Dad did not have to experience the physician's anger and feel alienation by the medical establishment. The social worker completed an impossible task in fact finding for the court system.

In follow-up: The orthopedic surgeon said the child should bear weight as tolerated. He explained that the child's bone will resorb and mold to the proper stress lines over time.

Reiki can reduce pain and stress.

On the case of the 12 year old with a pelvic fracture I quickly met my past, thanked it, and pressed on with my life. All with the help of Reiki.

CHILD ABUSE TODDLER
Sexual Child Abuse And Neglect
(SCAAN)

I place my hands for self-Reiki almost every night and often during the day. This regularity may be the reason I am less sad and fearful when thinking about my past than I used to be. During the Reiki I realize I am free from having to exist in the state of the abused victim.

However, as an earlier case attests, I am not perfect. I do not always remember the perfect state.

I was flying through the ER cases completing chart after chart and patient after patient in the Emergency Room (ER), being efficient, being Goddess of my ER territory on that day when the nurse said, "Dr. Eos, don't you think 3's reaction is a little unusual?"

'3' is the number of the room where a three year old patient and his mother were placed for a complaint of a swollen knee. The child had what appeared to be hives and mosquito bites over his whole body.

He also had swelling and increased heat over his right knee with no tenderness of the bones of the knee and no trouble kicking and screaming the whole time any person was with him in the room other than his mother. Yes, something was wrong. The screaming to this extent was not a normal

Remember self-Reiki.

Think about Reiki before entering the room.

reaction for his problems even at his age. I had refused to notice the discrepancy on the first exam of the child.

I heard him crying and screaming from way across the ER. I thought about Reiki before I entered the room. Before going fully into the room, I stuck my head in and acted funny. This usually makes a child laugh before I invade their territory.

I flashed my quick bright-eyes look at her twinkling with playfulness. This stopped his screams and got his attention for about five and a half seconds.

The next ploy to gain a shred of his confidence was to (1) enter the room slowly but with authority, (2) pull up the doctor's stool close to the child and mother - equidistant from each - and then to (3) talk to the Mom in soft, low, soothing tones about the child. I asked how her boy had been doing prior to coming to the hospital.

Again, I got some fleeting recognition for the try at peacefulness but the boy continued flirting with hysterics. He would calm down totally with Mom so I knew the screams were not all from pain. The screams were from fear.

While I received Mom's history, I observed the child without looking at him. Next, I trained my full attention on the patient. I looked him straight in the eyes — he looked away and screamed hysterically.

I placed my hands on his feet allowing Reiki to flow like a faucet. He settled for about thirty seconds then fought hysterically — physically. I eventually completed the exam of heart, lungs, ears, throat, belly and the very important knee. It was hot and swollen in the soft tissue over and above the patella. I noted some bruises. I shut down. My past was about to invade my present.

Place the hands on the hurting knee.

I wrote furiously on the chart, ordering antibiotics for the cellulitis, ordering an x-ray, ordering, ordering, ordering...

I did what was expected of an Emergency Physician.

My continued questioning of past medical history and other verbal probes for a child abuse case revealed nothing. A brick wall.

A crying mother. A screaming, crying child clinging to his mother and content only when in Mom's arms with no one else in the room. When the door was shut then the child was quiet, in a fetal position with his head up against the mother's breast.

Did Reiki do nothing? I had placed my hands on the child's knee allowing Reiki. The child kept screaming. The knee problem was not going away.

"I have found that Reiki always works."

Later, I discovered the child had been abused. What we were calling mosquito bites were probably cigarette burn marks. What good was the Reiki?

Reiki outcomes are not always as expected.

"Sometimes... I am unaware of the best healing for the moment; unaware of other alternatives."

My expectation was that Reiki was to work toward a specific outcome for the child and that I was not to feel the feelings from my past. Always and ever. Reiki the boy and Reiki me. That should be enough. However, I have found continuously that Reiki always works. Sometimes, though, I am unaware of the best healing for the moment; unaware of other alternatives when I am attached to the results. Often I feel the need for me to cure the physical problem presented. In this case I felt like a failure for not curing the knee of its swelling — within seconds. The super-person part of me felt like a failure because I began to feel the helpless victim state as my personal state. However, Reiki always works.

The Reiki of the chart may have been the reason why the nurse was able to shatter my lead-lined glass wall of emotions which plunged me into the child's world. This nurse who had just adopted a second child from a third world country in her effort to save the world by mothering a small part of it. This nurse who delights in telling of the ordinary daily milestones of her child's discovery of life in her home. This nurse who sews the small animal toys we give to scared children in the ER.

This nurse who became alarmed at the abnormal hysteria of the little patient in Room 3, who heard the screaming terror, who saw the bruises in the shape of hand and finger grips on the backs of each knee and the tops of his little three year old feet. This nurse who brought it in to my conscious attention and made me respond so that I said yes, I agree with you, there is cause for alarm, I will relook at his bruises.

Yes, indeed, they were consistent with thumb and finger prints. I filled out the state child abuse reporting form. I called the Protective Services worker. I told her about the bruises and where they were.

She asked if I felt the child had been sexually abused. I said the body bruises and emotional affect were consistent with that possibility. I said the bond was good between Mom and child and that there didn't seem to be any reason to disturb that relationship tonight. The child did not immediately have to be taken from his environment without a thorough investigation. She asked if I had performed an exam for sexual abuse. I said no. The mom had not come for that. I saw no reason to risk battery on the child for that exam at this time. The bruises were older than a day or two. They were yellowing. The worker said she would complete the Protective Service's visit to the home tomorrow. I said thank you.

So, I still hurt when a sexual abuse case comes to the ER. Even though I self-Reiki daily, I still whisk into avoidance and withdrawal when I can. Here I am a doctor, a lawyer, a Reiki practitioner... reduced to profound sadness... over a three year old

"Reiki... pulled me out of my personal agenda."

kicking child with bruises... bleeding internally in soft tissue... not even daring to bleed outright. I cry.

The nurses cry, too. And everyone in the ER... cries. But at least we are recognizing the problem and crying together. The Reiki in this case pulled me out of my personal agenda and toward working with the nurturing nurse in a community effort to help families re-establish loving relationships.

A DIARY ACCOUNT
Tooth Pain

As mentioned, I place my hands on myself for Reiki.

For example: I needed to get my teeth cleaned before I left for an overseas assignment. The next day the dentist worked on my only cavity. It was a deep cavity into the pulp of a molar. I rejected any local anesthetic because of profound hypotensive reactions in the past to the injectable medications. So I managed the pain with the help of homeopathic remedies, Reiki and mind control. I sat through all the dental work with no anesthesia.

The procedure was tolerable but about three hours later I experienced the most intense pain ever. I hurt.

Thank goodness I had the next two days, Tuesday and Wednesday, off work. I used the time to manage the pain. I pulled in other people to help with Reiki — Reiki practitioners and Reiki Masters. I took indicated homeopathic remedies. Slowly the pain receded. I worked Thursday and Friday without much pain. Saturday night the pain became strong again. Sometimes during the day and always at night I had such trouble with the tooth and gums that sleep was impossible. I tried Reiki, affirmations, analysis, remedies...

Reiki complements other healing methods.

I determined it was real pain with a psychological origin. It had to do with decisions, support of the decisions, fear, and ego. And yet, I could not make the pain go away. Even with a lot of Reiki. The more quiet and still I became, the more it hurt.

I reasoned that the pain must carry a very important lesson I needed to learn. However, I must be stupid because I couldn't figure it out enough to stop the pain. I hadn't found the key yet to stop my pain. The pain continued intermittently for two weeks while I tried to make it go away.

Meditation seemed to help the most but the pain became so great that I found it hard to meditate. Where was the lesson? Why couldn't I learn it? Why didn't Reiki take the pain away?

Reiki is not a magic pill.

Before the pain I had laughingly said, "What am I supposed to do with my life in Reiki? I may have to be socked in the face with the answer for me to see it."

So then began my tooth trouble.

I was in pain.

I became the pain.

I was a servant to the pain.

I did not dissociate to get away from the pain. It was painful to open my mouth and let someone else alter my decaying tooth. I recognized that I wanted guidance and help from a professional: the dentist.

In my physical body I was in pain. In actions I was in fear.

Pain, what is its reason? Purpose?

If life is to endure only pain — like my toothache — like child abuse — why nurture its existence? Is pain another illusion that I try — probably in vain — to tell myself this is a great lesson, an opportunity to grow? Why doesn't the Reiki take the pain away?

The pain was so bad in my tooth and whole left facial area that I was taking homeopathic acute remedies and swishing with Hypericum and Calendula tinctures every two to six minutes night and day. Yes, all night. The ritual worked except twice when I took flower rescue remedy which then gave relief for about twenty minutes. I placing my hands for Reiki of myself non-stop, 24 hours a day. The tooth area felt better when my hands were over the cheek. I took no narcotic pain relievers. I took no ibuprofen or antibiotics.

My mind dwelt on pain control, mind over matter, healing, why me, what is my lesson, why haven't I learned it yet, etc.

I had done all I knew to do to change the course of events. Events proceeded regardless.

My tooth was extracted. The dentist used only an antihistamine locally. I used Reiki placing my hands on my legs during the procedure.

After the tooth was out the pain immediately relented. Just a dull throb left. No more problem. Swollen throat, cheek, half the tongue from the irritation of the

Hands may be placed for Reiki during dental procedures.

antihistamine. No particular problem. The side effect of the antihistamine is sleepiness. No problem.

My friend drove me to her house after the surgery. I noticed a book about pain on her coffeetable. It was facing me as I came in. I avoided it, went around the table and rested on the couch. I slept for hours. When I awakened, the book was staring me in the face again. It was about pain. It said that pain is a gift. It said that pain is a gift that nobody wants.

I had a pain before the tooth was pulled. I had not wanted the pain. I began reading the book.

The author had spent most of his adult life in India treating leprosy patients. I read that the reason leprosy patients have so much trouble is because the nerves to their extremities do not receive notification of pain in the periphery well enough to avoid trauma. The etiology of the orthopedic problems of the people with leprosy is because they cannot feel pain.

Reiki does not take away a gift.

Pain is a gift for people to avoid hurting themselves. Reiki would not take away a gift. Leprosy patients don't have pain therefore they have more trauma more repetitively with more injuries and develop complications from the injuries.

So I spent the next two days and most of the nights reading that book, sleeping, thinking, and recovering from the antihistamine side effects — and allowing myself Reiki of course.

Pain is a gift. Even headache pain. My headache pain comes and goes with anger. It goes, however, much more quickly with Reiki. The same phenomenon happens with colds. Perhaps the reason I am getting fewer colds is because I recognize my separation anxiety, dare to feel it as soon as I get a sore throat, and then allow myself Reiki. Yes, I am more present in my feelings than ever before. I put my hands on myself regularly for Reiki.

The best healing is not always total relief from pain.

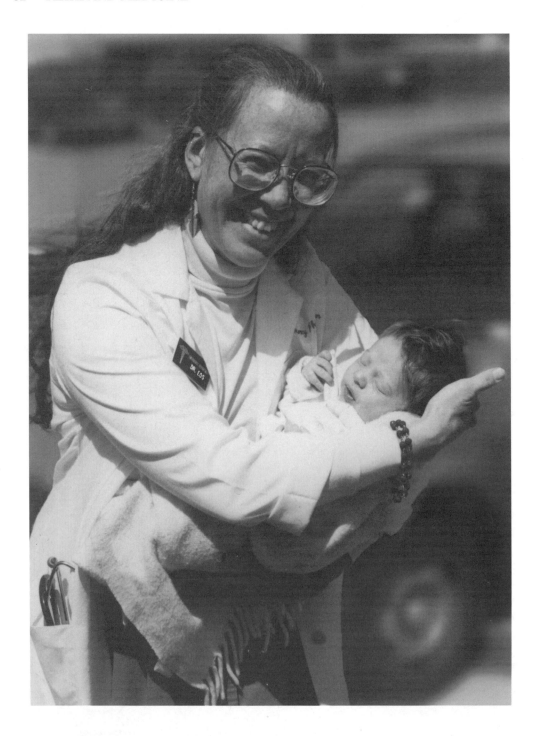

DIARY ACCOUNTS
More Cases

4 year old epiglottitis patient

One time I had a 4 year old with possible epiglottitis. After Reiki the diagnosis became subglottic narrowing which is a much less urgent problem. With epiglottitis standard medical protocol dictates that the child should be intubated by putting a tube down the throat to secure the airway before transport. With subglottic narrowing that is not a required procedure.

Always support Reiki with standard medical protocol.

The child came to the Emergency Room (ER) looking scared, sitting forward, with substernal retractions and drooling saliva from the corners of his mouth. I called the surgeon for a possible tracheostomy before transport. I called the anesthesiologist for possible intubation. I kept returning to the child every few minutes to place my hands for Reiki. By the time the others came to evaluate the child, he was better. They knew I did not usually cry wolf, though, so they attended the child in the ambulance to the pediatrics care center just in case something might happen enroute.

"I was able to see the Reiki results. His respiratory rate decreased just a tad, the lines in his face softened just a tad, he sat up straighter - just a tad."

The child did well.

Yet again, an invasive procedure was avoided.

Reiki often works dramatically.

"Immediately his countenance changed."

... a Reiki practitioner had used her fingers like a cautery unit to stop the bleeding.

23 year old male with pneumothorax

The weekend was hard work but all went well. One male was clutching his chest and having left lung trouble. He fell on a tree stump while preparing his tree platform for hunting. He suddenly felt better when I was listening to his lungs. He said aloud that he couldn't understand it. I did. It was the Reiki.

You should have seen his face — the changes were so obvious. He was hunched over and trying to position for that exact spot which might relieve his pain. He was not finding it. Before Reiki he settled on the least pain possible. I put my hands on his shoulder and asked him to tell me about the accident and the pain. Immediately his countenance changed. He began to half smile. Then he said, "Well... well... I think it is going away now." I smiled. I'd seen these changes before. Reiki was working dramatically again.

Bleeding thigh laceration

I had heard that a physician surgeon Reiki practitioner had used her fingers to stop some bleeding when she was in the mountain wilderness and had to perform emergency surgery on someone. So when I had a person with a big, deep, anterior, middle-upper thigh cut, I tried it.

It worked.

Complaining

As patients complain in the ER about what seem like trivial things, I place my hands on them, let the Reiki flow, and I invariably see them settle down. It is beautiful.

So I LOVE my hands.

"I love my hands."

Horses

I visited the horses one day. I felt one was sad and needed the homeopathic remedy Pulsatilla. I asked the stable worker if they used homeopathy. She didn't know what it was so I dropped the idea of mentioning Pulsatilla to the owner. I felt the horse was going to have trouble. My hands were very hot when I placed them on her.

Animals love Reiki.

I found out later that she was pregnant. Interesting. I had no remedies. I placed my hands numerous times to her neck for Reiki.

Months later I was told only one of the three folds from the three mares did well. Was it her? Interesting.

Cats and plants

I had my first set of Reiki attunements on a Saturday. On Sunday I placed my hands on my cat, my plants, and

Cats respond to Reiki.

Plants thrive with Reiki. After Reiki, cut flowers stay fresher- looking for a longer time.

two homeopathic patients. All are doing better than expected. Since Reiki, my cat looks more slim and trim and beautiful. My plants are green and lively. My house is airy and inviting... Little things. That's what calm is.

Parasites in food

Reiki enhances the taste of food.

When I was overseas, I placed my hands for Reiki over every meal and liquid passing into my body. All others eating the same food acquired parasites, some people were quite debilitated from the illnesses. I had no trouble and came home free of parasites. The Reiki? I'm convinced.

Electrocution case

Hands are for healing.

There was a 7 year old boy who had an arrest of his heart and his lungs. He was brought to the ER and was eventually fine. Moments earlier at a barn building he had touched some bare wires. He was thrown by the electric shock off a ladder onto the ground landing flat on his back. No pulse.

A chiropractor on the scene held the child's head in his hands before the Emergency Medical Services EMS unit arrived. The child began to revive.

I was impressed with the story. I also placed my hands ... for the Reiki.

The other ER Doc wanted to get a computerized tomographic CT scan of the head and other costly studies. The family did not want them. Also, they honestly felt the boy was going to be okay now. I did too. There were no signs of a deteriorating condition, only a remarkable history of significant trauma. I said I would release him without a CT scan. I took over the case and accepted legal malpractice responsibility. I trusted the Reiki. The child did well.

A typical night

One typical Friday night I had three unexplainable cases in a row:

(1) A 2 year old female with intractable vomiting came in her parents arms looking only mildly dehydrated and very sick. She looked bad. Reiki. I sent her to a bigger center. They sent her home less than 8 hours later. They found nothing requiring admission to the hospital.

Upset stomachs,

(2) A 14 year old male hit and run victim with a possible neck injury came by ambulance. Reiki. We transferred him to a trauma center. They sent him home that night. They found nothing requiring admission to the hospital.

neck trauma

and colic

(3) A 36 year old female health care worker with abdominal pain was brought by her husband. Reiki. She was watched by a surgeon all night. He found nothing requiring her to be taken to the operating room.

respond to Reiki.

Each case had many many positive findings for dire consequences. Statistically you would think that at least one of the three would have their condition evolve to needing more medical intervention than that.

"I place hands for Reiki on every patient."

I place hands for Reiki on every patient. Just a few seconds each time my hands are on. A minute is a luxury. If the patient is trying to code on me or have an MI heart attack, I stay right there for 5 or more minutes at a time. I try not to look too obvious. I just lay my hands somewhere on them — like their arm — and then talk to them or the parents or whatever.

Anger

The lines in their faces change as the Reiki begins to work.

I never have patients hit me now. They occasionally did before the Reiki. They must get frustrated at the process and by the time they see me they are angry and fighting. Then they hit. Now I begin Reiki for the situation before they get a chance to act out in violence. The lines in their faces change as the Reiki begins to work. Their anger disappears.

Addicts

Even addicts leave the ER saying "Thank you," as they leave. Even though they received no narcotics! I place my hands for Reiki to them, too. Our ideologies of what is best does not have to be the same for Reiki to work.

Blue girl

Next came a blue girl carried by her dad running into the ER. She was three years old. Since birth she was missing a lower chamber of her heart. She was blue because the oxygen was not getting into her blood stream. She was seizing. She pinked up instantly with Reiki. She began to talk. Interesting.

Reiki is simple.

The blue girl had aspirated. She does it occasionally. When she aspirates it blocks the windpipe and she can't breathe which causes her to become blue.

Her lungs were junky sounding on admission to the ER but they sounded clear by the time of transfer. She had vomited in the car while being brought to the hospital — usually pneumonia follows an aspiration of this type. It was a 40 minute ride from home to the ER — they came in 25 minutes. She was in status epilepticus — a very prolonged seizure state — but was calm after only a little Reiki and diazepam.

This was a very complicated case. Reiki, on the other hand, is simple. It is the simple things in life that count. There is no need to say, "Hold it everybody, I'm going to place my hands for Reiki to this situation."

Just place the hands in neutral territory for seconds to a few minutes and do what you would have done anyway.

No need to draw attention. No need to perform rituals. No need for acting. Just place the hands in neutral territory for seconds to a few minutes and do what you would have done anyway.

Questions

Later, I was talking to the paramedic who attended the man who collapsed at a store on the edge of our county. She asked if I thought it was Reiki that saved his life long enough for his relatives to say goodbye. I said yes.

Migraine headache pain

A practitioner has a Reiki energy field.

Something new happened last night. It may be an aspect of Reiki I had not considered before now. A 27 year old male came with a severe headache. He gets migraine symptoms often. Nothing but sleep makes the headaches disappear. He became scared this time because it had never before been so intense. He was without a migraine for two years. Well... on this visit to the ER he began to feel very strange when he approached the registration area. Then when I was in the examining room with him, he said he felt even stranger. The headache character changed. It was no longer painful. He just felt strange.

I had read something about energy fields which seem to surround us. Was he vibrating in my Reiki energy field and feeling it?

Even more strange, at the same time as he was being registered, I was feeling an intense tingle in my hands. The ER was quiet so I had retired to the Doctor's room. I was sitting reading when I noticed the tingle in my hands. I questioned what it might be. My hands continued to tingle. When I was called to the ER to see the new patient I again questioned why my hands were tingling. No patients were in route to the hospital by ambulance, there were no left over, incomplete, ER cases. I wondered if someone close to me were needing Reiki.

The tingle of Reiki in the hands is a background hum.

That's the other notation — I have slowly started to realize a slight nudging insistence to think about and Reiki certain individuals. I haven't had time to check out that sensation yet by testing it. I don't just believe in explanations of processes. I have to check it out as scientifically as I can. I was in academic medicine at one time, you know.

"I realize a slight nudging insistence to think about Reiki for certain people."

So when the 27 year old male headache patient was relating his story, I began to realize the tingle of my hands was not just a shout at a quiet me. The tingle was always present as a background hum. However, I rarely heard the hum against the shout of the demands of the ER. Interesting.

I like it when it is a bit slower and happenings may be analyzed a little more thoroughly. More may be noticed. The night shift is especially good for reflection of cases. Also, night people are a special breed. They seem to resonate at a different frequency.

Coughing child

One child came at the end of the shift. Coughing. Pulse oxidation metered at 89 percent. I let him go home after just one hour and many times of hands-on for Reiki. I reworked the case in my mind. Did the boy have Respiratory Syncytial Virus RSV? Was there another cause for hospitalization? Did I miss anything?

I called the Dad back after I got home three hours later. The child was better. No coughing. The nurses thought the child should have been admitted to the hospital.

Always support Reiki with standard medical protocol.

Am I going to overrate the abilities of Reiki some day and have to pay for it? I don't think so. I am very conservative. Standard medical protocols are followed — after a bit of Reiki. I wait for a change in the patient during the Reiki. A change that is not a normal course of events without the Reiki. These days I am brave and dare to use less aggressive conventional medical treatment and trust more to the Reiki.

ANAPHYLAXIS
A Total Body Reaction
and
The Physical Examination

It's fun to watch the human body and analyze its restorative workings. My mind's eye sees which system is working and how it is working. Observing the disease process affecting the person, I speculate as to what response is most efficient for that body to do when so stressed.

For instance, consider the course of an anaphylactic reaction which is a major allergic response. An example is a person allergic to penicillin who receives penicillin in their vein. I see these allergic responses as little irritating antigens of penicillin creeping into a body. Then I see the body's immune system take action. I watch a play of molecules dance around, collide with and attach to others. Then I see a feeling come over the patient by a change in muscular tension or relaxation. Then a rash appears. Then the sinking of the blood pressure begins. The tightness of chest, the fear, then eventually comes the attempt of the kidneys to clear the blood of the left over antigen-antibody complexes that were not able to deposit in the skin or elsewhere. Then with my mind's eye I see kidney failure, swelling and sometimes death.

When conventional medications are used for anaphylaxis, I enjoy thinking of the mechanism of action of the diphen-hydramine, steroids, and theophylline for

There is a usual course to most diseased or unbalanced states.

the reaction. I feel the need for hydration to dilute the responses. So intravenous fluids are given. The person becomes better right before the observer's eyes. That is fun.

It doesn't always work that way. Often, too often, the allergic anaphylactic reaction happens, the intravenous fluids are poured in, the diphenhydramine and steroids are given, the right responses happen, yet the patient crashes doing poorly.

The crashing is where I concentrated for a long time. It seemed the more I wanted and worked for a particular result, the less that particular result was the outcome.

"Science. I believed in it. I worshipped it. It was not working all the time."

I believed in double blind research. But I could never seem to control all the variables. As soon as I thought I had all of them defined so I could learn to control them; I'd see the problem in a different way. Low and behold — sure enough — up popped another variable to consider. I made too many confining assumptions.

I decided the way to be a perfect researcher is to define the arena — set limits — don't allow the project to go beyond those assumptions. That's what I had trouble with. Setting limits. No, the trouble is not in setting limits but in sticking to them. I set my limits well but then I would look at the patient and the limits would burst.

For instance — the asthma patient. I limited the patient to asthma. Well, I cured the asthma fine. And there would be NO indication of any other problem —

young, healthy, no other disease, no enzyme deficiencies. But — he would crash. Why? So off I would go again to try to get to the bottom of the intervening problem.

Didn't he want to be cured? Was the trigger still triggering? Were there side effects of my medications? Once I opened the limits to look at more variables, I often found a cause. The reason for the crash was different at different times. Then I began to wonder if I could ever get a hold on all of this ... scientific healing.

So I studied the philosophy of medicine. I continued to read a major scientific journal a day and a textbook a year. I tried psychic healing. I learned some energy medicine called homeopathy. I learned the philosophy and methods of homeopathic masters. At first I used remedies after conventional medicine failed. Then I introduced homeopathic remedies at the same time as scientific medicine during two years in a setting where I could use both in the ER. Then I began reaching for remedies while conventional medicine was ordered but not yet given.

At each step I watched the difference from the predicted conventional medical course of events. There was a difference. The results were toward a gentle and longer lasting change to body harmony. I worked, analyzing each step, until I could use the straight homeopathic remedies and see a cure before having to initiate the conventional medications. I was happy.

Patients often do poorly even though the standard medical protocol is followed.

"Using only straight, regular medicine in the ER would mean shifing thoughts and actions back to medications with side effects as the single choice to help heal."

Reiki is balance and rhythm in action.

Reiki penetrates objects.

Then, when I moved to a different Emergency Room (ER), I was told I could not use homeopathic remedies. I wasn't sure I could go back to straight, regular medicine. It would mean shifting my thoughts and actions back to reintroducing medications with side effects as the first line and only choice to help heal.

And I still had a problem with patient's attitudes. Many people I treated NEEDED their illness. They were not ready to be well. They had no concept of being ok in wellness.

So I had to contemplate going back to ER work without energy medicine. I went ahead and signed up for shifts in the ER. I needed an income. Economics are a part of the healing world.

My young-woman daughter was attuned to Reiki by a Reiki Master shortly before this. She was walking and moving through life with even more beauty than before she took the Reiki class. I researched where the new rhythm may have come from. It appeared to come from her experience with Reiki. I asked for Reiki on me.

She and a Reiki practitioner friend of hers twice placed their hands for Reiki on me. I was fully clothed. They put their hands on me. They talked when they wanted. They generally didn't seem to me to be doing a thing. I received no flashes of light, intelligence, good health, or other noteworthy thing. I just had a twitch in my left leg that later became a cramp. The cramp stirred up memories which broke a recent period of emotional memory distress. I was sure the string of events had nothing to do with the Reiki. Or did it?

After one month of returning to an intense ER without an energy medicine available to use, my daughter said her Reiki Master was coming to town. She invited me to the free introduction time the night before the classes.

I was curious about this Reiki method. I knew the energy healing process practiced by my daughter couldn't hurt. I had tried it as a patient. Reiki didn't interfere with other procedures like talking or thinking. So, I decided to jump right in and try it. During the evening introductory class I signed the list for Reiki.

I attended, received attunements and felt no different. Oh well, perhaps money down the drain but it was worth a try. It didn't hurt and it might help.

Since then, my whole life has changed... but I am getting ahead of the story.

Reiki does not interfere with other procedures.

I went back to work in the ER the next day. I had impossible patients. I felt I knew psychologically why they had their illness. Why couldn't they see it, deal with it and get on with their lives? For instance, knee and ankle strains were from fear of stepping out, hesitation, and unbalance. The patients didn't see this at all. They just hurt and wanted relief from their pain — maybe a cast and a narcotic.

"I found excuses to put my hands on the patients."

"I watched their facial lines and bodily stance change..."

The beauty of Reiki is that there is no special procedure. There is nothing to do right or wrong. There is nothing to 'initiate it' in the ER.

After attunement, get your hands on people and the Reiki will flow.

Allow the results to happen as they will.

So about midday I decided I would try this Reiki stuff. I found excuses to put my hands on the patients and I left my hands on the swollen sprain a few seconds longer than usual while I engaged the patient in conversation. I watched their facial lines and bodily stance change right before my eyes... the same changes I had seen when giving homeopathic remedies. These changes began when I placed my hands on the patient. I did nothing more. I was not the doer. I was merely attuned.

I searched for the truth of medicine. In giving in and giving up I found the truth. The truth is that my part in the play of medicine is to initiate a well meaning act and then allow Reiki — a universal life energy — to take over. I need to accept that we are all a part of the same life energy.

So, once attuned, after permission, get your hands on people and the Reiki will flow. Get your hands on the patient's back as you listen to the lungs with your stethoscope. Shake their hand and put your other on their shoulder. Get your hands on the hurting part. Then allow the results to happen as they will. Accept the highest healing good. You are not the doer. Don't demand results. Don't limit the patient to your wishes. Your belief system is limited.

The Trauma Exam

When a trauma case comes in, start at the head — or the foot. Place both attuned hands on the part. Look, listen, and feel all at the same time. Then move one hand further on the body, then the other. Stop. Look. Listen. Feel. First one hand change, then the other. Stop. Look. Listen. Feel. Touch every part. Assess. Assess. Assess. While your attuned hands allow Reiki, Reiki, Reiki.

No folderol.
No ceremony.
Once attuned,
place the hands for
Reiki.

Do what you have to do to remain within the parameters of standard medical practice: give orders, call specialists, and write in the chart. But don't think the results of the patient's healing is limited to that. Try Reiki, too. You'll find that if you allow for extraordinary events, they happen.

Always follow standard
medical practice.

When you get another chance, again place the attuned hands on the patient. Reassess. Reiki, Reiki, Reiki. Do your standard medical procedures while you allow Reiki each time you touch. And after the excitement — allow Reiki to yourself. Find the truth in what happened. You were not the healer but you were able to be a part of the scene. Then place your hands for Reiki again. Reiki, Reiki, Reiki.

You'll find that if you
allow for extraordinary
events, extraordinary
miracles happen.

Have fun with it. Reiki is freeing. Soar with it. Soar freely. Be in a Soaring Free state.

After the excitement...
allow Reiki to yourself.

Take the pulse

Feel the pulse. Instead of feeling with just the fingertips — find a way to wrap your hand around the wrist to feel the pulse and use the other hand to steady the wrist.

Reiki is freeing.

...wrap your hand around the wrist.

Get your attuned hands on anywhere, as soon as possible. Preferably while the patient is still coming into the ER. Especially when they are coming by ambulance.

Palpate the abdomen

Touch the elderly belly as soon as possible.

With older patients I go right over and touch their belly as soon as I can. I place my hands on top of the cover, the sheet or the hospital gown. Bowel function is very important to the elderly. Most doctors do not expend a great deal of time and effort in palpating their abdomen, — the most important area to the old person. So feel it. Not deeply, not hurtfully. Just place the attuned hands there, hold them there gently for a few seconds, and then feel around a bit. Allow Reiki to the elderly belly.

The Physical Exam

Hold the patient's head.

Hold the patient's neck.

My complete ER physical exam for ambulatory patients is three minutes long. I am able to initiate Reiki at the same time. I begin at the head, eyes, ears, nose, throat, HEENT exam. I hold their head with one hand and shine a light in the eyes with the other to see the pupillary response and look at their healthy iris. Next, I poke a light in each ear and look in the mouth. All the while I am examining, I place the free hand on the person's head. Reiki flows. After putting the scope away, I take their neck in my hands to feel for lymphadenopathy. I hold my attuned hands there a little longer than necessary while I allow the Reiki to begin. I usually ask the patient a question to distract them a bit while I allow the Reiki to work at the neck. Sometimes I feel the sinuses or forehead for more Reiki to flow.

Hold the patient's back.

Then I move the attention to the back to check for spinal tenderness. I place one hand on their shoulder closest to me. The other I place at the base of the skull, feel the cervical spine then touch and gently push each vertebrae while moving my hand down the spine. Instead of using my fingertips, I place as much of my full flat hand on the spine as possible. I use the base of the hand as a steady fulcrum for the fingertips to push the part being tested for tenderness. To check for costovertebral angle CVA tenderness, I place one hand at the right or left costovertebral angle, pause with it there, tell them I am testing for kidney trouble then hit the hand with my other fist. The flat hand is allowing Reiki.

Next is to listen to the lungs. I place both attuned hands flat on the back and manage to get my stethoscope head between the fingers somewhere. I listen as long as I can while I think Reiki, Reiki, Reiki.

Place both attuned hands flat on the back.

I leave one hand on the back while I take my stethoscope to the chest area to listen to the heart. As much as possible and without touching senitive areas, I try to lay at least part of the hand out flat around the stethoscope head.

Hold the patient's hands.

Hold the patient's shoulders.

Hold the patient's knees.

Rest your hands on the belly.

Touch the forearm.

The process of allowing Reiki looks no different than a normal exam.

Next, I perform the neurological exam. I ask the patient to squeeze my hands, pull arms up against mine, down against mine, then shrug up against my palms which happen to be placed on each shoulder ... Reiki. Then I place one hand on a thigh near a knee while checking the deep tendon reflex DTR's with the other. Then I keep the one hand near the knee and use the other to grasp the heel. I passively check for full straight leg raise by raising the heel to a 45 degree angle to the spine. I test the other leg. This allows Reiki on yet more joints.

I ask them to lie back. When they get settled, I place both my hands on their mid-belly. I rest there to settle the hands while in my mind I am thinking Reiki, Reiki, Reiki. Then I palpate the abdomen. The whole process of allowing Reiki looks no different from a normal emergency physical examination.

To let the patient know when I am finished, I place a hand on their forearm, or shoulder, or lateral leg or whatever seems safe for the patient and tell them they may sit up. Again touching. Again Reiki.

The complete exam is almost always done with the patient fully clothed. I don't want to invade privacy. I don't want to invade. Even if I am to do a pelvic, I do the above exam first. Then when the patient is undressed and in a gown I again go over parts of the exam before the pelvic. Reiki and Reiki before invasion.

CONCLUSION

I want to tell each person touched with Reiki, "I'm glad to have known about you and your ways." I want to ask how each is doing now at one, two, and three years after the Reiki. How each is living life.

Was there a decision on their part to die, not die, continue disease, become healthy? I hope the touch of Reiki during their emergency was a breather for them to regroup and redirect their health. That is all that I ask.

Theories are just that — theories. Perhaps the truth of medicine, the art of healing, will never be known. In scientific reality, we have no perfect explanation as to how or why Reiki works. It just does. And that fact is what is important to me. Theories and ways of coming to the energies of healing are important but... I prefer to just let the Reiki be. No folderol. No ceremony. No attention getting acts.

Personally I prefer the unadulterated Reiki with no explanation but that — it works, try it.

Pain is not present to be endured. I don't believe that it is necessary to suffer in order to learn lessons. It is not necessary to suffer in order to work. Pain is a gift. Listen to the message from your body. Pain is to be recognized and heeded for its warnings. Once on that path of realization, that pain may be placed aside by any method including Reiki that works for the patient.

My walk with Reiki has literally taken me to Mountains, Plains, Deserts, and Valleys. My walk has been around and past every individual I have known. It has taken me through life and death, pain and pleasure, happiness and grief. My whole life has changed. And yet, sometimes, it seems that only the emphasis has shifted. Perhaps the syllables of my song are still the same but the shift in accentuation has changed the whole rhythm and meaning of the song.

Every patient became a discovery with Reiki. Besides just placing the hands on the patient — I concentrated on having Reiki available for the patient earlier and earlier. Besides absent Reiki to the territory covered by the hospital Emergency Room (ER), I tried to catch each person as they entered the trek to the hospital.

Then I waited for feedback. It came.

People would say things like, "I began to feel better just entering the doors of the Emergency Room."

Often it is not that dramatic. Like last night.

A 76 year old male came in with shortness of breath. He was an escalating chronic obstructive lung disease patient from smoking who will soon need to be on home oxygen. He had increasing shortness of breath and wheezing over three days. He over-used his inhalers.

What did I have to offer him from the ER? —only a nebulization of the same drugs that hadn't helped all day. The latest double blind studies show that whether the drug is delivered by hand inhaler or nebulization doesn't matter. In fact, the nebulizer treatment has been declared to be unnecessary. The directives came down in the last ER memo to give hand held puffs instead of the expensive nebulization. This patient had already overdosed on hand held inhalers. And he had them all.

So I placed my hands for Reiki as I talked to him. I put my hands on his back to feel for rattling. Then I listened to his lungs with my stethoscope keeping my hands flattened out over his chest and back. I would alternate being intense on listening and then talking making light of something.

I was able to see the Reiki results. His respiratory rate decreased just a tad, the lines in his face softened just a tad, he sat up straighter — just a tad.

We hooked up the nebulizer for the breathing treatment and before it could begin to work he commented on how much better he felt. I made a reference to the nebulizer saying how great the treatments are. He looked at it, lit up, smiled and said yes. He was looking for an explanation for the change. I gave it to him. He was satisfied. Scientifically there was no way that the treatment could have been the answer to his healing.

Patients seem to be that way — often. Incredulous at a change for the better. They look, sometimes frantically, for an explanation. If they don't get one they often relapse back a little. When one is provided, they become serene, the change settles in and health may even progress a little bit.

It is so much fun these days to treat people. I love being a doctor. I am learning a lot about myself.

I hadn't realized how scared I was doing emergency medicine until the fears were gone. I didn't realize how hard I was trying for an impossible perfection in emergency treatment until I saw the irrelevancy of one person's efforts to change another person's course.

Note, I did not say that a doctor or nurse or healer does not matter. I said that the effort or degree of it is irrelevant. It is the love that is relevant. Take away all medicine and healing except love and note that the results are not only as good, but better. No side effects of a nature that is detrimental to the health of the individual.

The fact of nurturing has been well known forever. But I overlooked it in my modern medical training. For years I tried hard to attain an objective, scientific perfection of conventional medicine and dispense it with a side salad of psychic healing, new age healing, and pity. I worked hard to manipulate the bad illness of the patient and make him well. I wanted to make the hurt go away by my active killing of the pain for the patient.

Well, Reiki has changed my whole life, my whole way of approaching healing. I no longer heal. I go in and out of people's lives, touching theirs, allowing a universal energy-love to be taken or not taken by the person in dis-ease with their life. And I am happy. No fear. No performance on my part to be fearful about. There is an acceptance on my part. I accept that the person has this illness as a means of working through whatever he needs to get wherever he is going. When the person consciously or subconsciously accepts their part in a universal oneness, the knot unknots, the illness and dis-ease with their life in this body dissolves into health.

And the part that I am is observer ... to see myself. My own remaining dis-ease to resolve into health.

Questions and Answers

What is *Reiki*?

The *rei* aspect of Reiki means unlimited, air, universal, boundless, spirit. It is the cosmic principle of energy.

The *ki* aspect of Reiki means energy, power, life force, vital. It is the denser daily life principle of energy.

The rei and ki of **Reiki** (pronounced "RAY-key") when together means unlimited energy flow between matter and energy. Perhaps much like the concept of $E=mc^2$. Energy may be converted back and forth into and out of matter when related to a relevant constant. Perhaps Reiki is a facilitator of the conversion.

To complicate the simplicity with theories is to bind Reiki to limits. Many teach/give it without explanation. Some teachers superimpose their interpretations of energy healing or spirituality.

One theory is that the Reiki practitioner focuses a time and space for interaction of 1. a cosmic transcendental inner energy with 2. other kinds of physical or mental energy much denser in vibration.

Reiki is simply an unlimited energy flow from the universe through the hands of the attuned practitioner
> ...unless you unbind even this.

One aspect of Reiki is a form of hands-on-healing I have used on myself and on my patients. It is Love. It is quiet. There is no need to alter consciousness while using Reiki. Reiki goes through a person as if the person is a conduit. Unlike a conduit or tube, a Reiki practitioner can become Reiki — a Reiki practioner can become a balance and harmony of unlimited energy flow.

The key to this special knowledge of the power of healing through the use of the hands was preserved in Sanskrit. A formula to the key was discovered. The formula is in a series of symbols which, when set into motion, activate and tap universal energy.

How do I receive *Reiki*?

Request it; honor it; receive it — as a practitioner or as a patient. You can consciously or unconsciously accept the gift of Reiki.

There needs to be an exchange of energy. It is not right to be indebted for services rendered. It is not right to indebt others. The exchange need not be money. The form of energy may be in a trade. If the person requesting treatment or knowledge is a family member or very close friend, a normal exchange of energy is already taking place continuously.

How do I learn *Reiki*?

Ask a Master for attunement;
Honor the time/energy/knowledge;
Receive the attunements;
Use it: Reiki, Reiki, Reiki.

If I don't use *Reiki*, can I lose the ability?

No. Once attuned, you have it for life. The energy does not become exhausted. It expands with use but you must use it to benefit from it.

You can't use Reiki wrongly.

Reiki always works
                    ...but it may not produce the outcome hoped for.

What is the Usui system/lineage of *Reiki*?

The Usui system of Reiki is the working knowledge of Reiki as rediscovered by Dr. Mikao Usui and built through the direct lineage from Dr. Usui to Dr. Chijiro Hayashi to Mrs. Hawayo Takata.

This Reiki knowledge is transferred from a Usui system Master to a person who offers a sacrifice for the gift. The transfer is by way of attunements. The attunements are in stages. The traditional stages are:

1. Reiki I
2. Reiki II
3. Master

It is best to take Reiki II at least 3 months after Reiki I. Three years is suggested for the Master level.

What is *Reiki I*?

Reiki I is the basic *Place the hands, allow the Reiki to flow*.

This is enough. There is nothing more that is needed to practice Reiki.

Reiki I involves receiving four attunements or energy transfers to align and fine tune the chakras or energy centers. These attunements are by a Reiki Master.

What is *Reiki II*?

Reiki II accentuates Reiki I. It includes *Reiki from a distance*.

In Reiki II one learns more teachings and receives more attunements. The attunements are by a Reiki Master.

In Reiki II one learns some of the ancient symbols used by Dr. Usui.

What is a *Reiki Master*?

A Reiki Master is Reiki all the time. A person becomes a Usui Reiki Master by dedication and commitment of their life to Reiki. Being a Master is not a business or profession. A Master is something one becomes. When one chooses this life style a period of intensive study is monitored by a Reiki Master who trains and initiates Reiki Masters.

What is the 21 Day Settling Period?

Some Masters feel that the first 21 days after an attunement is a cleansing period. It is suggested that the new practitioner do at least 20 minutes a day of Self Reiki during this time. Keeping a journal of experiences is helpful.

What are the Five Principles of Reiki?

Just for today, do not worry.

Just for today, do not anger.

Honor your parents, teachers and elders.

Earn your living honestly.

Show gratitude to every living thing.

ORIGIN IN LEGENDS

Dr. Mikao Usui

The origin of Reiki is steeped in legends traditionally passed in the oral manner. One belief they have in common is that Dr. Mikao Usui was a great being who rediscovered Reiki while reading the original Sanskrit Buddhist Sutras in the late 1800's. The telling around this story varies. The following includes some of the common points.

Dr. Usui was a Christian minister, scholar and professor in a small Christian university in Kyoto, Japan. One day a student challenged the teacher to demonstrate what he taught. The student asked:

If you believe in the healing of the sick by Christ and his disciples using the power in their hands, demonstrate it today.

Dr. Usui had absolute faith in the Bible. He believed in the healing of the sick through the hands. Was it blind faith?

The question sparked a need for more knowledge. Unable to answer the needs of his students, Dr. Usui resigned his position that day. He went in search of the answer for how the hands can heal. He first came to the United States where he obtained a doctorate degree in scriptures with top honors from a university in Chicago. Still no truth of enlightenment for his question.

Dr. Usui kept his faith. He searched other philosophies. He found that Buddha had also used the power to heal with the hands. Dr. Usui returned to Japan to study with the Buddhist monks. Most monks explained to him that their focus was on healing the spirit, not healing the body. Physical disorders are left to doctors of the body. Dr. Usui kept his faith and kept his question. He continued the search.

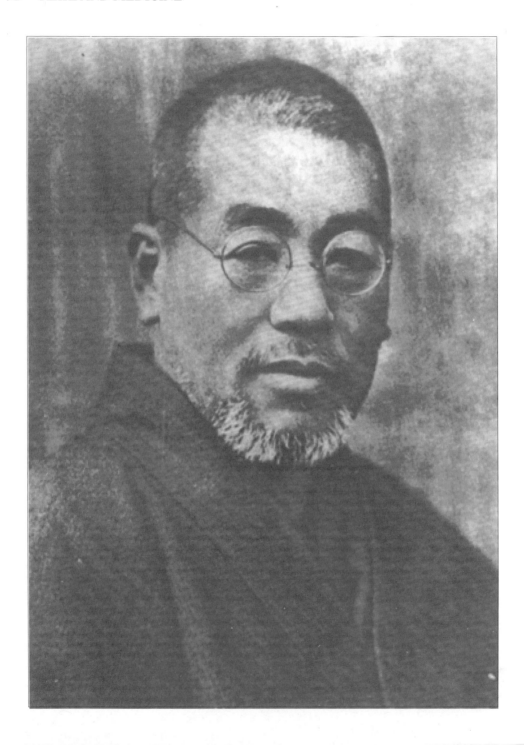

At a Zen monastery he was refused admission until he repeated the five spiritual principles. He repeated them as he knew them.

Just for today, do not worry.
Just for today, do not anger.
Honor your parents, teachers and elders.
Earn your living honestly.
Show gratitude to every living thing.

He studied the Japanese translations of the Sutras. After learning Chinese he studied the Chinese translations of the Sutras. Then he learned ancient Sanskrit and went to India to read the original Buddhist writings.

In them Dr. Usui found the answer. He found the description of how Buddha healed.

Dr. Usui thought he was finished after 7 years of searching. For seven years Dr. Usui put his total self into the search, kept the faith, and found the answer. But he felt he was not ready to use the knowledge. He spoke with the Buddhist abbot from the Zen monastery. They decided he should go to a mountain to meditate. He climbed a sacred mountain of Japan to meditate for 21 days. As each day passed he set aside one of 21 stones. On the last day a light came and swept through his consciousness. He saw the keys for the answer he had discovered in the Buddhist texts in bubbles of light. The keys to the healing by the hands used by Buddha and Jesus was burned into his being with the light.

There were then four things which displayed the Reiki:

1. Even though he had fasted having only water for 21 days, he felt rejuvenated and energized.
2. He stubbed and tore his toenail while running down the mountain, grabbed it with his hands and the wound was healed within minutes.
3. Where he stopped for food a woman with tooth pain asked for help and was cured when he cradled her face in his hands.

4. As he talked to the abbot and rested his hand on the old man's shoulder, the abbot's arthritis disappeared.

The next seven years Dr. Usui worked healing the sick in a beggar camp in Japan. He set many of them up outside the camp with food, clothing, and a job. One day he noticed them returning in the same condition as before they were cured of their disabling diseases. He had healed one part, but not all parts of the people. A life change had not occurred from within the person.

The next seven years Dr. Usui wandered day and night with a lighted torch. He began to teach only others who wished to know how to heal themselves. He gave them the Principles of Reiki to help heal them wholly.

Dr. Chujiro Hayashi

Dr. Chujiro Hayashi was a retired Naval officer who met Dr. Usui and asked for the knowledge of healing with the hands. He stayed and continued to study with him. Eventually Dr. Hayashi founded a clinic in Tokyo where people came for treatment and to learn Reiki. He documented with records that Reiki finds the source of the physical symptoms, fills the vibration or energy need, and restores the body to wholeness.

Mrs. Hawayo Takata

Mrs. Hawayo Takata went to Dr. Hayashi in 1935 from Hawaii. She was to have surgery in Tokyo but was treated with Reiki for about eight months instead of having the operation for her tumor. After demonstrating a commitment to Reiki, she was trained over three years to the Master level. Later, Dr. Hayashi named Mrs. Takata his successor in the linage. It was Mrs. Takata who brought Reiki to the United States.

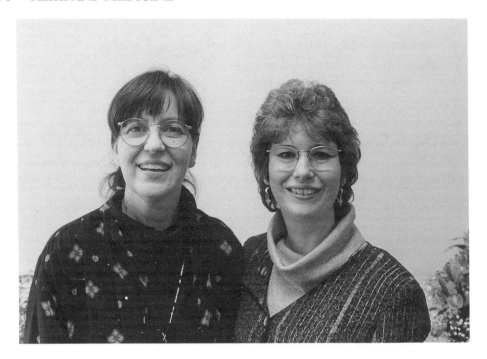

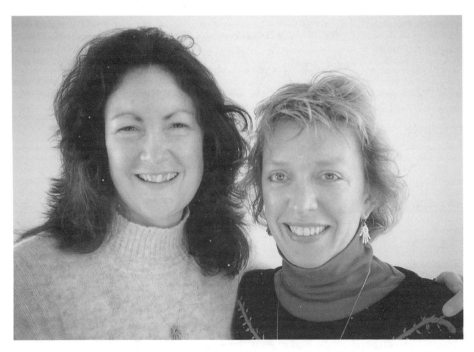

Reiki Masters

There are many *Reiki Masters*. We support one another. Some of us in Michigan are: Mimi Becigneul, Anna Gagern, Nancy Steel, Suzy Wienckowski, and Nancy Eos.

Some *Reiki Masters* giving classes and working in pairs are:

Mimi Becigneul, DCSW, NCTMB, and *Anna Gagern*, DCSW, NCTMB
     17117 West Nine Mile Rd., Suite 419
     Southfield, Michigan 48075
     810-569-5430

Nancy H. Steel and *Suzy Wienckowski*
     4548 Breezewood Court
     Ann Arbor, Michigan 48103
     313-668-8071

Libby Barnett, MSW, and *Maggie Chambers*
     RR #1 Box 212
     Wilton, New Hampshire 03086
     603-654-2787

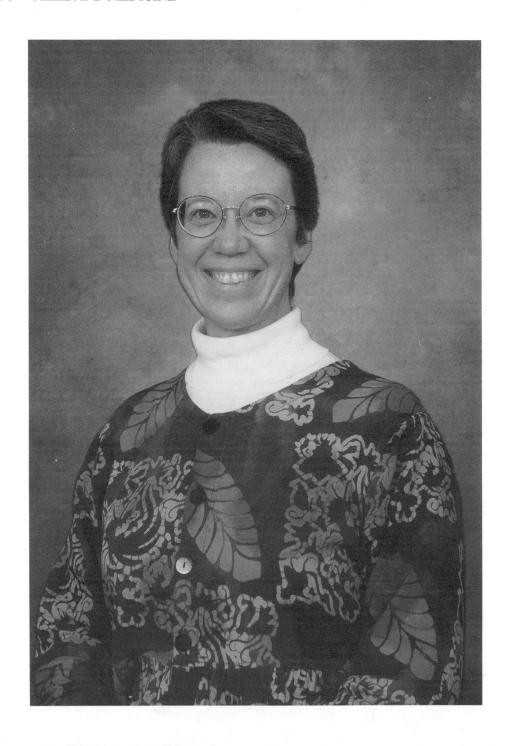

BIOGRAPHY
NANCY EOS, M.D.

Dr. Eos practices family medicine at Grass Lake Medical Center in Michigan. Reiki is an integral part of her medical practice. She is also an educator for Reiki and Homeopathy.

1968 Bachelor of Arts; Oakland University, Rochester MI
1973 Premedical studies; University of Rochester, Rochester NY
1978 Medical Doctor; University of Michigan, Ann Arbor MI
1990 Juris Doctor; Thomas M. Cooley Law School, Lansing MI
1991 Arizona license in Homeopathy
1994 Reiki Master Initiation

Dr. Eos' children Heather and Sankey were in grade school while their mother was in medical school. One weekend the three of them were driving between Ann Arbor and Ypsilanti. There was an accident just ahead of them. Dr. Eos stopped, jumped out, and began CPR on a non-breathing driver. She looked up to see her children's faces in full wonderment watching her. It brought a close bond between them of understanding about health care.

In the 1980's Dr. Eos was a part of the teaching staff of the University of Michigan Medical School, University Hospital, Ann Arbor, Michigan.

She is author of *The PREP Book: The Physician's Rapid Emergency Peripheral-brain Book,* a handbook of drugs and groups of drugs for emergency physicians, and *Survival Flight* an autobiography.

Other speaking engagement topics include (1) *Sexual child abuse* for the Federal Bureau of Investigation in Nevada and Court Appointed Special Advocate CASA volunteers in Michigan and (2) *Homeopathy* for the United States Public Health Service, Indian Health Service hospital staff in Arizona, Nevada, and South Dakota.

Dr. Eos served in the United States uniformed services as a Lieutenant Commander in the Commissioned Corps. She was Director of Emergency Services on two isolated American Indian Reservations.

She volunteers as a physician on third world country projects overseas and mountain trail restoration service trips in the Americas.

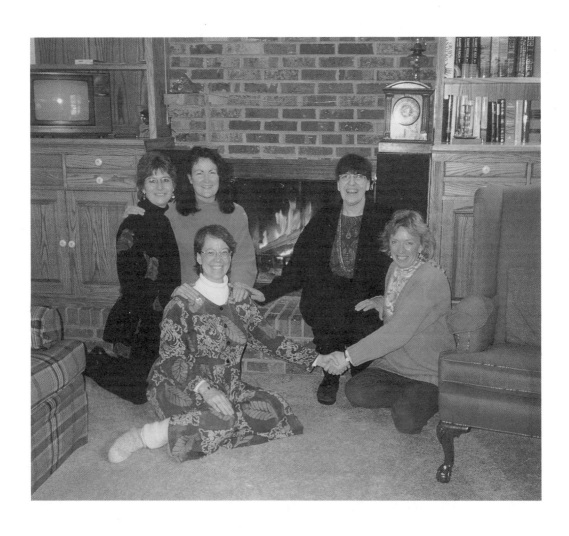